Stress At Work

Stress At Work

A study of a growing problem
in industry

Rowland Goodwin, B.A. B.D.,
D.M.S.

Chester House Publications
2, Chester House, Pages Lane, London N10 1PR

First published July 1976
© Rowland Goodwin, July 1976
ISBN 0 7150 0063 2

Printed in Great Britain by
Cox & Wyman Ltd, London, Fakenham and Reading

DEDICATION

To my father
ALFRED HENRY GOODWIN
Foreman dyer
and cancer victim;
the human cost
of whose work
could never be repaid.

ABOUT THE AUTHOR

Rowland Goodwin is a Methodist minister working with the Teesside Industrial Mission in the North East of England. He was born in 1929 near Warrington, Cheshire, the only son of a farmer's daughter and a foreman dyer. He was educated at Urmston Grammar School and served in the Royal Army Medical Corps during his National Service. After demobilization he worked as a farm labourer. He entered the Methodist ministry in 1950. After a period in Carlisle he studied at Manchester University where he graduated in 1954. He was awarded a further degree by London University two years later. He has spent most of his life in working-class areas. He had a close association with the docks in Bootle before moving to Bristol in 1956. His father died in 1960 as a result of contracting cancer of the bladder at work. He spent five years in Lanarkshire, Scotland, where many of his contracts were in the engineering and steel industries. In 1965 he became one of three men appointed by the Methodist Church to work full-time as an Industrial Chaplain and has lived throughout a period of radical industrial and social change in Darlington. He is an honorary member of the Darlington Trades Council, Chairman of the Darlington Careers Association and, in 1973, gained a Diploma in Management Studies at Tees-side Polytechnic with a distinction in Personnel Management.

He is a frequent lecturer at Luton Industrial College and is married with three teen-age children.

FOREWORD

Some years ago, I invited the Rev. Rowland Goodwin to make a special study of the very important subject of Stress at Work. In the ensuing years he has lectured on the subject at various courses held at the Luton Industrial College. On every occasion he has been a great help to members of those courses and the people present have been drawn from a very wide field of human activity, including managers, trades unionists, college and university students.

The author has brought to his subject a mind well endowed with intellectual qualities coupled with a desire to serve men and women as they seek to live a whole and purposeful life in contemporary society.

Much has been said in recent years about change, but we have yet to realize that the rapidity of change is now taking a heavy toll of human personality.

The technological explosion has caught men and women off balance. We are clever enough but can we cope? In all the hurry of modern life can we create mental open spaces in which we can reflect? Are we capable of adapting ourselves to our rapidly changing environment?

The Governors of the Luton Industrial College express their gratitude to the author for accepting their invitation to write this book as a College Foundation Lecture commemorating the historic event of the opening in October, 1976 of the very considerable expansion of the college buildings.

Further, we express our gratitude to Chester House Publications for making this publication possible.

William Gowland,
Principal, Luton Industrial College.
July, 1976.

CONTENTS

		Page
	Foreword	7
	Acknowledgements	11
	Introduction	13
Chapter One:	The Stress Problem	17
Chapter Two:	What Causes Stress?	31
Chapter Three:	What is Stress?	36
Chapter Four:	The Stress Symptoms	44
Chapter Five:	Stress Levels	50
Chapter Six:	Stress Patterns	56
Chapter Seven:	Stress at Work and in the Community	61
Chapter Eight:	Stress and the Supervisor	71
Chapter Nine:	Allen's and Brown's	76
Chapter Ten:	What can be done about Stress at Work?	114
Conclusion		130
Questions for discussion		133
Reading List		135
Appendix A	Table showing the correlation between Job factors and stress	137
Appendix B	Certified Sickness Absence-year ending June, 1974	138
Index		139

ACKNOWLEDGEMENTS

I am deeply indebted to the Principal of Luton Industrial College, Bill Gowland, for inviting me as far back as 1970 to take part in a course on middle management. The background research which I had to do for this produced much of the material contained in the first chapter of this book and it made me aware, for the first time, of the growing problem of stress at work. Groups of managers, trade unionists, student teachers, clergy and others have since used my input to that course which was printed by the College under the title *An Exercise on Stress*. The document has been also used by a number of firms and in supervisory training programmes in the North East of England.

In 1972 an opportunity came my way to make a much more scientific study of the problem of stress at work and I am grateful to the members of the staff of the Management Department at Tees-side Polytechnic for helping me to undertake a detailed project among four groups of supervisors in two contrasting companies. This project formed part of a two-year course for the Diploma in Management Studies which I was awarded in 1973. I received secretarial as well as tutorial help without which this project could not have been completed. The late Dr. G. O. Hughes, Chief Medical Officer for the North West Gas Board, gave me invaluable help in working out a suitable basis for the measurement of stress levels; a critical part of the whole exercise.

I gave an undertaking to the men and women who took part in the research that I would not allow anyone but myself access to the questionnaires which they completed for me nor would it be possible for anyone reading the report of my findings to identify any one person. I have kept to that pledge in this book. Any name that appears is quite fictitious. But I would like to express my appreciation to all those who shared in the work and to the managements at both companies who gave their permission and showed so much interest. I felt it wise to call the two firms, Allen's and Brown's.

I am also very grateful to the manager and staff of the Print Room and Typing Pool at Cummins Engines Limited, Darlington, for doing work for me at both the project and book stages of my study.

Many other people have expressed interest in the research. I am indebted to Dr. Alexis Brook, Consultant Psychiatrist at the Tavistock Clinic in London and to Dr. Joseph L. Kearns, Medical Adviser to the Joseph Lyons Group of Companies for their encouragement and helpful criticism. This has led me to rewrite certain sections of my original manuscript.

The Managing Director and staff of Crompton Lighting Company Limited, Doncaster, gave me the opportunity to conduct a Stress Analysis among a cross-section of personnel. The lessons I learned from this exercise have helped me in my approach to other companies.

INTRODUCTION

This is not a highly technical book. It is written mainly for those who have stress situations at work and are aware of the problem but need help in understanding what stress is, what causes it and what might be done to overcome it. This book is one person's attempt to put down on paper a number of industrial situations as he sees them in the hope that others may recognize familiar circumstances and be encouraged to do something positive about reducing stress levels before more serious and damaging consequences develop.

This book is not a 'last word' on the subject. Far from it. Stress is a very diffuse and complicated subject. It has to do with human beings who, in themselves, are complex creatures. But these complex creatures operate in a wide variety of roles; being, at one and the same time, a partner in a complex web of domestic relations, a subject of government and a worker by hand or by brain. It is often difficult to know whether something that looks like a symptom of stress is actually a symptom or a cause. There are so many variables – personal factors, family difficulties, workplace pressures, cultural influences – acting on any one person at any one time that it becomes virtually impossible to untangle any one situation and say, with any overwhelming degree of certainty, 'There, that's the root of the problem.' One may well doubt anybody's dogmatic statements about human stress.

This is part of the problem about tackling stress at work. It's not as simple and as straightforward as many of the problems managers and men are trained to handle. To launch into a stress project is, for many, to enter into a dangerous exercise. We lack understanding, confidence and competence. If one tries to take into consideration all the factors which could conceivably react together to produce a stress situation one might well be put off taking any action at all. Meanwhile, the longer nothing is done, the worse the problem gets. In the working situation it can result in the collapse or death of key personnel. Almost certainly a company with a stress problem will suffer reduced efficiency, and lost productivity. The cost of doing nothing will rapidly begin to exceed the cost of getting somebody in to handle the situation. This is the dilemma in which some find themselves at work.

This book is, therefore, not a comprehensive study. The basic research that sparked it off was structured deliberately to exclude a wide range of personal, domestic and cultural factors in order to concentrate on the working environment. Within this working environment the book relies heavily on work done on one small, but significant, section of one occupational group. Here are just a few snap-shots of what a researcher found. Much more work will have to be done before anything like a whole scene emerges. But, just as a few pieces of a jigsaw puzzle can give a clue to a wider view, so this book is offered as a contribution to a clearer understanding of stress at work, how it can be identified and assessed and what might be done to prevent problems getting worse. It is this latter issue that presents greatest difficulty.

No one reading this book must make the mistake of believing that reducing stress levels and increasing job satisfaction or a sense of well-being at work is either easily or cheaply attained. Some things, as the reader will discover, can be put into practice quickly and with the minimum of cost and result in immediate benefit. But the solution to the stress problem at work lies more in the direction of wholesale redesign than in piecemeal adjustment. In this respect the changes taking place in certain Scandinavian companies have tremendous significance. Nor must it be assumed that either the problem or the solution to the problem can be devolved on to one group, be it medical, employer or union organization. Just as each bear a measure of responsibility for allowing stress situations to develop so each share responsibility for creating less stressful working conditions. Very few of the problems identified in Chapters One or Nine could have been solved by taking a bottle of tablets and a fortnight off work. The offering of, or the demanding of, extra money to compensate for work that leaves a man irritable, depressed and alienated is no adequate solution. If solutions are to be found they will come as a result of co-operation and joint action between all interested groups.

If this book can help stimulate a determination to reduce stress levels, if it can prompt further research into and understanding of stress problems and if it can encourage the coming together of resources which, apart, have no chance at all of reducing stress but which, together, might have some success, then the effort involved in writing it will have been worth while.

ROWLAND GOODWIN

Darlington, 1976

Chapter One

THE STRESS PROBLEM

Stress at work is commonplace. Anyone who is caught between conflicting pressures at work will be able to talk about stress either in himself or as he sees it in people around him. It is more acute in some occupations than in others. Assembly-line workers, caught between the moving track and what appear to be the insatiable demands of the employer, know what stress is, or, if they cannot clearly recognize the beast, they are aware of its presence. Supervisors, who find themselves often standing between what management must have and men don't want, are particularly prone to stress problems. Accountants, who struggle to hold a working balance between cash flowing out of the company and cash flowing in, know what stress is. Senior executives, watching the activities of competitors, weighing the effects of fluctuations in market forces and witnessing inefficient companies going to the wall, will have little hesitation in listing situations where they and others around them have been caught in a stress problem. Stress has become part of life. Just as overtime has been allowed to establish itself as part of the normal process of getting things done in some industries, so stress, potentially dangerous though it is, has become an acceptable consequence of work. In an industrial society, caught as it is at a point in history of rapid and radical economic, social, technical and organizational change, stress problems may well worsen until new attitudes and new systems can be developed to control them.

A flurry of literature in the 1950s and early 1960s by men such as Russell Fraser, Elliott Jaques, Hans Selye, Frederick Herzberg, Georges Friedmann and others was the consequence of considerable interest in the effect of the working environment on mental health. Herzberg, writing in the preface to his book, *Work and the Nature of Man*, said that industry must realize that it is one of the despoilers of man's efforts to achieve happiness – in spite of management's most sincere attempts to do just the opposite. 'For the first time in history,' he argued, 'we have the opportunity to satisfy man's inherent wants. Yet what value to man if industry manufactures commodities to supply material comfort at the expense of human development and happiness?' At the time of writing, in 1966, Herzberg regarded mental health as 'the core issue of our times'. Although evidence exists to show a steady growth of stress at work, interest since that time has, if anything, declined. Research into the effect of the working environment on mental health has been limited. In Britain, a special committee was set up under the chairmanship of Lord Alfred Robens to look into the matter of Safety and Health at Work. Its findings were published in a two-volume document in 1972. Nowhere in the publication was there a sign of concern for the stress problem, despite the fact that evidence was submitted to the committee by the National Association for Mental Health. The Act of Parliament which followed the committee's work came on to the Statute Book on the 31st July, 1974. It was equally reticent on the subject. Significantly, though, its title was changed from *Safety and Health*, a traditional industrial ordering of priorities, to *Health and Safety at Work*.

While month-by-month figures of fluctuations in employment are published by the Department of Employment in Britain and days lost from work through industrial disputes are watched with fierce intensity by Press and public alike, the minimum of publicity is given to days lost through mental ill-health. In 1970, when the Trade Union Movement began its campaign against the Government's proposed legislation on Industrial Relations, over ten million days were lost from work through strikes of one kind or another. It was the first of a number of bad years. On the Continent Frenchmen and Germans referred to 'the English disease'. British industry and the British economy were sick. Indeed they were. In 1970, according to information produced by the Office of Health Economics, a private concern with headquarters in London, a total of thirty-six million days, three times the amount of days lost through strikes, were lost through mental ill-health. But these figures received little publicity. In fact, if truth could be told, the situation was much worse. The total of over thirty-six million was arrived at by counting up the days recorded by the medical certificate system; a process by which employees off work for more than three days obtain a certificate from a doctor and send it to their employer. A true picture of days lost from work through mental ill-health would have to take into consideration casual absence; the odd day or two days taken off here and there. But, even this figure, as a measure of stress at work, would be inaccurate. Only when one takes into consideration the reduced efficiency and the lost productivity by people still at work but unable to give of their best because of anxiety or fear or depression or indecision or any one of a score or more symptoms by which stress shows itself can the full impact of the problem be grasped.

The Office of Health Economics showed that mental illness, over a thirteen-year period, emerged as the second fastest growing cause of days lost from work. It claimed more working days than influenza and the common cold put together and more than the whole range of accidents.

Attempts to estimate the cost to industry of stress at work have been both limited and fragmentary. In the United States a study of alcoholism has produced a figure of £4,500 million as the estimated total cost to industry. Equivalent British costs are put at £500 million a year. Looking at the problem as a whole one cannot doubt the truth of a headline which appeared in the *Financial Times* on 28th April, 1974. It read, 'Stress costs more than strikes'. The full cost must be enormous.

There are human and social costs as well as the efficiency and lost productivity costs of industry. A co-ordinated system does not yet exist in Britain to help the person under stress. It is there in parts, but fragmented. Medical treatment of ill-health has been oriented towards the patient. Not enough attention has been paid to the influence of the working environment on a man or woman's health and sense of well-being. The medical profession, management and trade union officials have combined well together on the problems of men at work in hazardous and unsafe conditions. But the limitations of the work of the one thousand five hundred Appointed Factory Doctors at the beginning of 1970 are openly admitted in the January, 1974 issue of the *Department of Employment News*. 'The majority of AFDs spent only a relatively small part of their time dealing with industrial health matters, in which they have limited functions: the routine examination of young people entering Factories Act employment; the carrying out of the periodic medical examination of people working in hazardous trades covered by the

Factories Act regulations; and the investigation of gassing accidents and notifiable industrial diseases.' It is clear that there is not sufficient understanding of the problems of stress at work or, as yet, adequate liaison between the groups that might effect a cure if they could find a way of working together.

All too often it is the symptoms and not the root causes that have been treated. Where the patient in the doctor's surgery has been suffering from a problem of a largely personal nature some success has been achieved. There is no doubt that in this kind of situation the medical profession has a major role to play. But where the causes have been largely to do with the working environment, requiring radical job redesign or organizational change, the lack of response from management and unions must have nullified many attempts by the doctors to effect a cure by the prescription of a course of drugs and a fortnight off work. The treatment that tackles the symptoms and bypasses the root causes can only have limited success. Likewise, as Herzberg has shown, money, paid out in compensation for soul-destroying work, will only buy short-lived satisfaction. Ever-increasing wage offers and wage claims are no satisfactory solution to the problem of stress at work. The lack of money to purchase essentials will certainly cause stress; the thick roll of bank-notes at the end of the week will not necessarily produce happiness.

To earth the problem of stress at work in some kind of reality the remainder of this chapter is given over to a description of a number of real-life situations. Frank, Edgar, Colin, Alex and the rest exist. Only their names are changed. Each one is a different person speaking out of a unique set of circumstances. Resolving their stress problems may well require individual help as well as job redesign and organizational change. This poses yet another problem. How good we are at the technical hitches. How quickly we can sort out the production bottlenecks. How incompetent, insensitive and lacking in confidence we are in the one-to-one emotional relationships.

Stress will never be eradicated from work. Influences exist outside work into which no boss or shop-steward, however sympathetic, has a right to pry. But it ought to be possible to do something about the working situation which these men describe in order to reduce the stress and lessen the industrial, social and personal costs which are invariably its consequences.

Frank

Frank was rarely in his office when you wanted him. He had the kind of job that took him everywhere about the works. Today, the office door was open. I was in luck. At his desk, behind a pile of papers, sat Frank. I knocked and stuck my head round the door. 'Come in. Won't be a minute.' He scribbled away, making notes on a pad. Inevitably, the telephone rang. He answered it, spoke, put the receiver down. It rang again. Frank grimaced and cussed. Problems, problems. But that was Frank's job. In a couple of minutes he was finished. He sat back. 'Well, what can I do for you?'

He was obviously very busy and under considerable pressure. The tension showed in his face. I wondered whether to go on or not. I chanced it.

'I can see you're busy, but I need your help, Frank. I've been asked to take a couple of sessions on "the pressures of middle management" at a conference in about a month's time and I want some short, thumbnail, case-studies to back up what I want to say. I can come back later if it would be more convenient, but I would like your views about stress if you can find the time to talk to me.'

His response was immediate.

'You've come to talk about stress?' His face was alight with interest. The clatter of typewriters and the incessant ringing of telephones in the main office sounded through the half-open door. 'Just you sit down there and let me shut that door.'

Frank talked to me for the best part of an hour about his work. He outlined how his attitude to his last job led directly to the breakdown of his first marriage. He talked about his current problems and his attitude to work. He described in vivid detail a typical day's work; problems with planning, problems with material shortage, problems with machine breakdowns, problems with the people directly responsible to him and those for whom they were responsible, and, all the time, pressures from above.

'Can I share a problem with you?' he asked.

'Sure,' I said, 'go ahead.'

Swivelling round to his right he lifted up a mat that lay on the polished-topped drawers behind him and drew out a sheet of paper from underneath. I thought it a queer place to hide correspondence. In fact, it wasn't correspondence, but a list of strengths and weaknesses of one of Frank's men.

Frank explained how serious the situation had become in a key area. It was a problem that had to be resolved without much more delay. There were many contributory factors, but, primarily among them, was the attitude and competence of the man Frank had tried hard to understand. It was more than likely that he would have to be fired.

'It's been on my mind for some time,' Frank confessed. 'I know a show-down has to come, but I've kept putting it off, hoping that things would improve, but they haven't. I've got to see him either tomorrow or the day after and I'm still not certain about the best way to approach him. I was awake most of last night thinking about it.'

I knew the person concerned quite well. Together, Frank and I talked about the advantages and disadvantages of the choices open to him. We came to no definite conclusion, but Frank said it had helped to share the problem with someone else. We agreed to keep in touch. I felt that I had seen a man under considerable strain and was grateful to Frank for being willing to talk. I thanked him and got up to go. As I turned at the door to say, 'Cheerio,' I saw Frank slide the sheet of paper under the mat.

I never saw him in his office again. The telephone rang next day and I learned that he had been rushed to hospital with a thrombosis and was dangerously ill.

It was sometime before I was able to visit him. I found him confused and incoherent. I waited for an opportunity to mention the paper under the mat, but the right moment never seemed to come. Some months later Frank came back to work, but although the company tried hard to rehabilitate him, he never recovered sufficiently to take up his old job again. Frank's 'problem', meanwhile, had left the firm and I never was able to discover the precise circumstances that led up to his departure. Frank, himself, is now working elsewhere.

In the weeks prior to the conference I interviewed twenty-five people. By the time the talks were due I had plenty of evidence about stress at work.

Edgar

He was in Production. The pressures on Edgar at work were very heavy. He found it difficult to stop thinking about work even at home. He kept a note-book on the table beside his bed. Often, after thinking about a particular problem, he would drop off to sleep, only to wake up at two or three o'clock in the morning, still turning the problem over in his mind. The notebook was handy for jotting down ideas. When I talked to him he looked on the verge of nervous exhaustion. He admitted to being under stress. He put his problem down to having to produce parts more quickly than the system allowed, in an environment of continual change, a total lack of foresight by management and poor planning.

Colin

He was part of a Sales team. His problem was that there was too little time within which to achieve objectives. According to Colin, it wasn't just breakdowns in the Production Department that caused problems, but failures in human relations. He was afraid of the effect of the pace of life on his health. 'At work, the pack rushes off and you go along with it,' he said. 'In the social race you are like dogs in the traps and, from "the off", the leader sets the pace.' The stress problem was made worse because he found it difficult to see any link between the basic values in which he had been brought up to believe and the kind of life he felt he was being forced to live. 'It's like having to do a thousand-piece jigsaw puzzle,' he said, 'with pieces being fed to you one at a time which don't fit.'

Alex

'You've caught me at a good time,' said Alex. 'I've got an ache in my neck and jaw right now. It always comes when I'm under stress.' He certainly looked flushed and tense. He was under pressure from several different sources and struggling also against time. He confessed that worrying about the financial situation at the firm made him lose a lot of sleep. Alex felt that it was impossible to forecast every difficulty. When there was plenty of cash around it wasn't so bad, but when money was in short supply things were much worse. Frustration built up for him, on realizing, after the event, what could have been done to save the company money. He described his job as 'juggling with plates spinning round on the end of sticks with some falling off'.

Martin

Like Alex, Colin and Edgar, he, too, was struggling against the pressure of time. His problem was not just to achieve production targets but to do so in a way that pleased the Boss, the Unions and the Sales Department. He felt he was in an impossible situation; trying to be fair to different groups with different, and, sometimes, conflicting interests. What bothered Martin most was that while trying to be fair himself other people were not only unfair to him but inadequate and dishonest. Nor was the problem just a work problem; society as a whole seemed unfair.

Scott

Scott's job was to recruit employees in order to meet labour requirements in the different departments of the works. His major problem, at the time, was one of redeployment. It was being made worse for him by two factors. One was the difficulty of getting decisions from senior management on requests made by those requiring staff and the other was the unreasonable criticisms by departmental heads that the lack of response to their requests was due to the sheer inefficiency of the Personnel Department. Scott complained that not only were decisions from above slow in coming but some of the refusals for additional manpower were turned down without any reasons being given. This made relationships particularly difficult. Scott complained of recurring headaches. They always came on at work. They mysteriously went away at home.

Len

He was at a higher management level than Scott. He saw the difficulty some companies had to survive in an economic environment which called for organization, efficiency and quick responses to changes in legislation, trade, financial liquidity, new business policies and ethical concepts. Len felt that the setting of goals was causing pressure for many British managers because, for the first time, they themselves were being measured against challenging objectives. While Len did not appear to be under stress himself he did admit to the difficulty of handling the masses of information that poured into his office. He believed that the situation would get worse. Another problem was that people did not know how best to manage a group situation nor were they all that willing to allow others to help.

Ben

Stress was a very real factor for Ben. He recognized it in himself and saw it rubbing off on others. As his own work slowed down so did that of his secretary. There were times when she had nothing to do. Ben felt that underwork was just as much a stressor as having too much to do. He faced a situation at work where there was continuing disagreement between people, a regular backlog of work and an inability to fulfil job requirements. Another problem Ben faced was the inability of people to communicate or put into effect what they, but no one else, knew they wanted to do. Stress at work affected relationships at home. Ben said he tended to treat his wife's comments as 'moans'. Because he did not listen always to what she said he did not hear or appreciate the points she was trying to make.

Louis

A fairly placid person himself, Louis also was aware of stress. Panic spread quickly in times of stress. It was his experience that people were most vulnerable in off-periods, especially if they were under pressure to produce results by an allotted time. 'They become one-track minded and withdrawn so that you can't get anything out of them.'

Vince

'Frustration builds up in a production area,' Vince said, 'when, having made a plan and gained commitment to it, machines break down, the plans are lost and new ones have to be made.' Often breakdowns were outside anyone's power to control. Person-to-person conflict occurred in his area every half-hour. It was the nature of the job. Job apart, Vince's main source of stress had more to do with an inner conflict about the purpose of life. He didn't see work as the main purpose at all. He felt that what he did outside working hours was far more important. This caused problems because Vince found it a struggle to motivate people to achieve objectives at work when work no longer was a prime motivation to him. This caused distress, worry, indecision. 'I dream of being sacked', he commented. He felt it was a problem only he could resolve but he was uncertain about what to do for the best.

Ralph

Working with computers meant, according to Ralph, being subjected to intense pressures from many sources. Working in small teams sometimes complicated matters. Relationships tended to be strained when people did not get on well. Operating under a three-shift system when there was a shortage of trained personnel created extra work-loads, bigger demands, greater pressures and more problems. Ralph could tell when people were under stress; there was a marked deterioration in accuracy and a falling-off in performance. For himself, he was conscious of being irritable and short-tempered at home and, over the last couple of years, had dropped out of a lot of social commitments.

Jeremy

He was in no doubt at all about the problem of stress at work for managers. He saw its source both in home and business life. Very often, the two were in conflict. Jeremy's business life was one of searching out for orders and short delivery schedules. As a senior executive, he felt it was becoming increasingly difficult to survive. Costs were important in the face of competition and increased efficiency often called for redundancies. It was an environment within which companies could not afford mediocre managers. Old companies, under the stress of commitments, monthly programmes and outside pressures were particularly vulnerable. Many of them were going to the wall. A shortage of competent managers could cause a man, perhaps with little ambition, to be thrown into a situation where he felt right out of his depth. The consequence of pressures at work showed in over-work, ulcers, stoppages in promotion and inability to delegate.

Neil

Neil's problems stemmed more from domestic worries than from work, though, like so many others, he commented about the difficulty of getting through priorities in the time available and the increasing tempo of working life. He felt a continued tension between family and work responsibilities. Concern about ageing parents, a wife in the middle of a change of life and problems over teenage children increased this tension. Neil felt it was not possible to give up family responsibilities or easily shrug off domestic worries at work. With a previous wife he had put her interests first. This had stopped his promotion and, now, he felt some resentment. Having to deal with people at work with similar problems to himself only exacerbated the situation Neil felt himself to be in.

Gilbert

He was one of the people who found himself thrust into a situation at work where he felt competent in one half of his job and much less so in the other. He had been propelled into his job when one of his colleagues recently left the company. Customers were pressing for deliveries. There was a back-log of work. The new situation had been stimulating for a time, but, now, a crisis wasn't far away. Part of Gilbert's feeling of stress, he felt, was self-imposed. He set high, perfectionist, standards both for himself and for others. He did not find delegation easy. He wasn't keen to admit his deficiencies. He had difficulty in responding to change. Under stress, he found that his mind locked-up. Dull aches and numbness developed. Tablets and tranquillizers gave only temporary relief. His capability and effectiveness were affected. He found it difficult to avoid thinking about work when he was at home. A spell in the garden or wallpapering a room didn't help matters either. He applied the same perfectionist standards at home as well as at work. His wife had problems also, being on her own all day. Gilbert was clearly worried. Was the ache a result of stress or was it the sign of a brain tumour he wondered?

Arthur

Deciding the priority of jobs was one of Arthur's main problems. Pressures came at him from so many sources. At holiday times, when there were so many staff shortages, he often felt unable to cope. 'Even though I'm normally placid, I begin to boil inside, especially if someone comes along with a job that is not really urgent and they say, "Arthur, do this for me as soon as possible." Pressure develops in my head and I blow my top. Other people hear me and go away saying, "Blimey, things must be bad."'

Russ

Russ felt that Industrial Engineering was a potential stress area because it involved industrial relations between shop-floor workers and management. Although he said he was not under stress himself he said he did see evidence of it and felt that some people did not appear to realize how quickly it could build up. He had his solution. 'When I get a headache,' he said, 'I shut off.'

Max

He worked in the Drawing Office. Max had a theory that the more intelligent you were the more likely you were to become a stress sufferer. He traced his stress problem to conscientiousness and sensitivity. 'Conscientiousness,' he said, 'leads to workload and work-load leads to stress.' He went on, 'If someone calls me stupid I am affected for the rest of the day. I am ultra-sensitive; a real self-critic. I could kick myself all over the place. And if someone questions my loyalty to the company, this causes stress too.' Max said that at times like that he became withdrawn and found it impossible to be open with the person who was being critical.

David

His chief concern was Systems. At work he believed that knowing what the end was, or, as he put it, 'being able to see daylight at the end of the tunnel', helped him to cope with stress. 'If you can't see the daylight, and if nothing is being done to minimize stress, then, more stress is created.' He felt that stress was linked with the state of one's mind and with age. Young, hard-working people, he felt, often felt the need to be frank but were apprehensive about rocking the boat too much. David talked about a particular domestic crisis that had caused him great stress. 'It was made worse because I could not analyse my feelings at the time and I felt uncertain about the feelings of the family towards me.'

Bernard

Bernard summed up his situation as follows: 'You come to the office with five objectives in mind but you are not able to get round to any of them because of other work waiting, a queue of people, the telephone, answers required on problems that are not really immediate. On your own level people resist pressure, so there is a tendency to go around and above people in order that pressure can be exerted by someone in higher authority. This may get things done but it builds up pressure and causes resentment and stress between colleagues.' Bernard felt that one could be under pressure without realizing it and the hectic life could be interesting until, as he put it, 'one external pressure tips you'. One problem he had identified about himself was his readiness to make himself available to all people at all times. This caused stress. Another problem was his inability to delegate. He loved to be involved. The consequences were that correspondence did not get answered, work was not done on time, frustration built up through failure to reach objectives, headaches developed, then migraine. At home the wife would say, 'I've never seen you this week.' She was able to sense the stress, but could not understand the cause.

Adam

Adam travelled about a lot. He put his stress problems down to fatigue, inter-personal conflict, the inability of managers to work as a team, failures in communication and having, from time to time, to take decisions which hurt others. Like Bernard, he made himself available. 'I never refuse to see anybody and I like doing good turns. But, by going after someone else's problems, I finish up with too many commitments. I set high standards and stress comes through trying to keep too tied to a schedule.' Loss of temper was one of his stress symptoms. His secretary said, 'Do you know, the minute he opens the door I know whether he is under stress or not.'

A group of six senior managers all agreed that stress was a factor of industrial life. One used the word 'skintight' to describe the management situation in his company. Reductions in staff, in order to cut costs and improve efficiency, had resulted in some people being loaded with responsibilities beyond their ability to cope. Under such pressures a lack of training and the opportunity for training were being revealed. In this kind of situation decisions were being taken on the basis of inadequate information and experience and this created sour situations which, in turn, produced more anxiety, fear and indecision.

Another member of the group, a managing director, spoke of the stress produced by take-overs. People began to look over their shoulders, he said, at others coming and going and began to be afraid of redundancy. He added that increased size did not automatically result in improved efficiency in every case.

The works manager of a small company commented on the heavy responsibilities borne by a few in charge of small firms and the consequent stress that that can produce.

It was generally agreed within the group that most compromise causes stress. 'At the end of the day you have a decision to make. You know it is not the one you would like to make, but circumstances, and the fact that you cannot easily give up your responsibilities, force you to make it.'

Frank, Edgar, Colin and the rest were just a handful of people picked, more or less, at random out of a number of management contacts. Statistically, their evidence would not carry much weight. What are twenty-five people among so many? But it was significant that everyone of them recognized the fact of stress at work. They saw its effect working out not just in their own lives but in their relationships with others and in their and other people's ability to get things done. There was some evidence of a confusion about the nature of stress. Some talked of pressure, others of stress. But there was no doubt that the problem existed and that work was one of the main stress-producing areas.

Chapter Two

WHAT CAUSES STRESS?

On the basis of the evidence so far presented there would appear to be four major stress-producing areas: the Workplace, the Personality, Industrial Society, and Home and Community.

What were the Workplace stressors for Frank, Edgar, Colin and the rest? It might be worthwhile to list them: conflict between people, departments and groups; machine breakdown; communication breakdown; inadequate systems; poor planning; lack of foresight; failure to reach objectives in the time expected; inefficiency; backlog of work; shortage of staff; too great a work-load; too small a work-load; unrealistic targets; mediocre management; incompetence; skin-tight manpower situations resulting from attempts to cut costs; lack of proper job definition; management politics; resistance to change; interference; compromise; lack of training and lack of opportunity to train; pressure from Sales; pressure from Production; pressure from the Boss; pressure from the Unions; pressure from Customers.

Undoubtedly, there are many more stressors at the Workplace, but these were the ones the interviewees identified.

The Personality stressors were as follows: acceptance of responsibility beyond the ability to cope; responsibility suddenly thrust on one without the opportunity for adequate training and preparation; inability to delegate; unwillingness to accept help; inability to develop good team work; inability to understand personal and group behavioural problems; hyper-sensitivity; perfectionism; setting standards for others and for oneself which are too high; failure to come to terms with oneself; having to compromise; lack of motivation; over-ambition; under-ambition; worry; resistance to change; lack of foresight; indecision; inability to handle masses of information; inability to cope with increasing complexity; insecurity; apprehension at being measured against a standard; inability to communicate; inability to leave work problems at work; uncertainty about the attitude of others; becoming too involved in other people's affairs; inability to please the Boss; fear of dismissal; fear of redundancy; lack of openness; loyalty to the company; ill-health; loss of effectiveness; lack of achievement; conflicting beliefs.

The interviewees commented about stress 'rubbing off on others'. They listed other stress symptoms such as tension, anxiety, withdrawal, loss of temper, depression, fear of health breakdown, overwork and the debilitating effect of headaches, muscular aches and migraine.

Stressors in Industrial Society were also identified. These were: pressure from competitors; financial pressure caused by fluctuating rates of exchange, shortage of cash, price variations; changing business objectives; rationalizations and redundancies; redeployments; labour shortages; mergers and take-overs; pressure from social or consumer groups; company failures; impact of new technology; the impact of new business methods; new legislation; complexity; accountability; necessity to compromise and the changing pattern of industrial relations. The more senior a manager is the more likely he is to be aware of such factors.

Not least were the Home and Community stressors: tension between husband and wife; the family versus the firm; concern over teen-aged children; concern over ageing parents; pressure to keep up with the social race; uncertainty about the meaning and purpose of life; the influence of marriage breakdown; the effect of putting one's wife before one's career; the inability of a wife to understand the cause of her husband's stress; the inadequacy of medical treatment that only treats the symptoms and gives but temporary relief; insufficient leisure; the pressure of social commitment.

In terms of quantity Personality factors came first, followed by Workplace factors, Industrial Society factors and Home and Community factors.

There would appear to be considerable evidence to support a view that, generally speaking, an attack on the problem of stress based on overcoming workplace problems could have a very beneficial effect on the nation's health and well-being. An individualistic approach, on the other hand, would have to identify the most dominant stressor, and this could be any one of a number of factors. These factors could well have little

What Causes Stress?

connection with work. Many variables, in fact, could be influencing a person's stress pattern. Some obvious. Others hidden. Some might be within a person's reach. Others might be right outside it. An expensive programme aimed, say, at improving work satisfaction, could help many. Others might not be touched at all because the main source of stress could lie in an area where no company, however well meaning, has a right to pry.

The question: 'What causes Stress?' has not yet been answered. Frank, Edgar, Colin and the rest identified factors which contributed towards a stress problem. Taken person by person factors which caused stress to some were not stress factors to others. The threat of redundancy, for example, might make most people anxious. For some, particularly those who have been through the experience before, it might be a welcome means of getting hold of a useful sum of money. One man's poison may be another man's meat. One set of circumstances may throw a man into utter confusion. The same situation may be taken by another as a challenge and lead to high job satisfaction and enjoyment. One cannot always determine how people will react when problems are put in their way. Everything depends on a person's ability to cope, and ability to cope depends, to a large extent, on the reserves of mental and physical energy that can be called upon in an emergency. Stress signs are most likely when the reserves are low.

The Energy Cycle of a person who works for his living is shown at Figure 1. He expends energy, physical and mental, at work. He has periods of relaxation during working hours; tea breaks, meal breaks and time off for a smoke and a chat between tasks. By the end of the day, or the shift, he is, nevertheless, tired. It is a healthy tiredness. He leaves the factory and heads for home. If the traffic isn't too thick on the road he begins a period of relaxation. By the time he gets home he may well have lost any tenseness he might have had at work. After a meal, a wash and a shave and a change of clothes he is ready for a few hours recreation. It may be at home, in front of the television, or out in the garden. It may be at the pub, with, or without, his wife, or fishing, or church, or one of a variety of leisure pursuits. But it is what he wants to do. It is recreational, and, even though it might involve some quite hard work or thinking, he enjoys it. At the end of it he is ready for bed. He and his wife kiss Goodnight, drop off into a sound sleep and wake, in the morning, refreshed and ready for another day. That is how it should be; relaxation, recreation and sleep, restoring energy expended in work. In reality, the pattern of the day is often quite different.

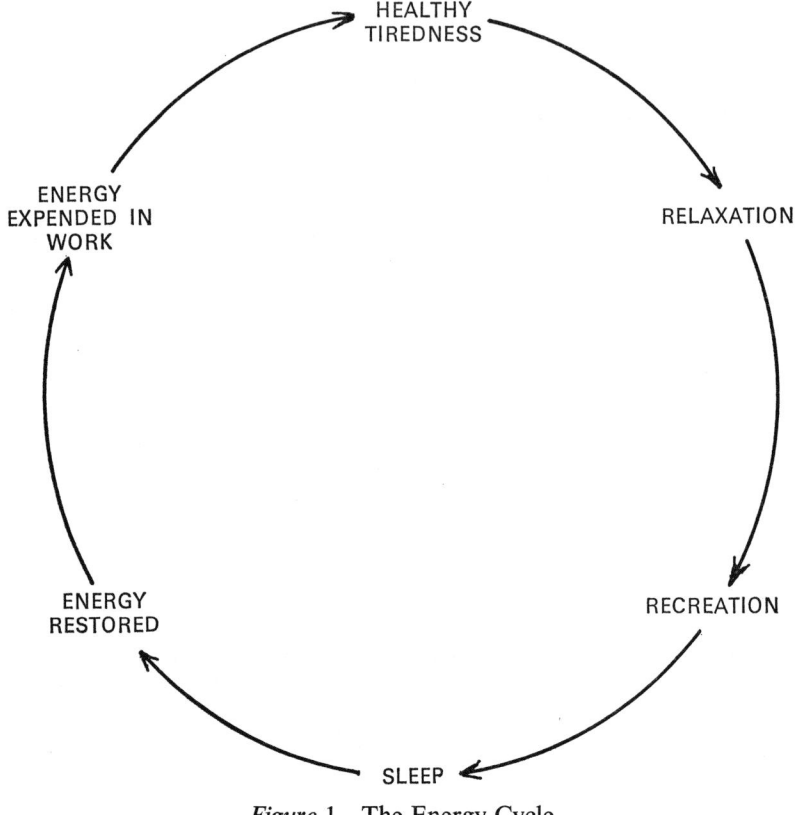

Figure 1   The Energy Cycle

Pressures at work may be such that although coffee comes in the morning and tea in the afternoon more than half of it is left in the cups to go cold. Meals may be hurriedly bolted down. Half an hour before the end of the day the boss may ask for an hour's overtime. After more than double the time the work may still not be complete and on schedule. Some folk have to leave so papers are stuffed into a briefcase and work is taken home. The drive is quick because there is less traffic about and the relaxation time that one would normally expect is all that less. At home an irate wife produces an overcooked meal. Husband escapes into the front room partly to finish his paper work and partly to dodge a tirade of complaints. By 10.30 p.m. exhaustion has set in. The wife goes to bed in a huff, her whole evening's plans having been spoiled by some dictator at the works who appears to have more control over her husband than she has. Bed-time eventually comes, but sleep doesn't. The baby wakes everyone up. The time: 2.30 a.m. By seven o'clock when the alarm goes off no one feels like stirring; no one, that is, except the dog who barks to be let out. The bitter dregs of yesterday are still with the husband as he drives, breakfastless, back to work. Over the twenty-four hour period there has been no relaxation; little recreation. Sleep has been fitful and broken. Another day begins with reserves in the energy bank at a very low level; hardly enough to take a man through a day when the boss is going to complain about work not being done on time. At sometime during the day, perhaps after what, to an onlooker, appears to be a very trivial matter indeed, the stress signs begin to show and the emotional temperature shoots up a good ten degrees.

What caused the stress? Was it the boss who pushed his men too hard and too far? Was it the man who failed to give himself time for relaxation? Was it the wife who, fighting for her husband's time, succeeded only in adding more pressure at the end of the day? Was it through lack of sleep? Was it the 'trivial matter' which, under normal circumstances, would have been ignored, but, on this day, pushed the man beyond his ability to cope?

It was all of these, and more. But, without the work overload, the stress might never have happened.

Chapter Three

WHAT IS STRESS?

The Oxford Dictionary defines stress as 'constraining or impelling force', an 'effort, demand upon energy'. In the mechanical sense it is 'a force exerted between contiguous bodies or parts of a body'. It is interesting to compare this definition with that for the word 'pressure', a word that is frequently confused with 'stress'. Pressure is 'the exertion of continuous force, force so exerted, upon or against a body by another in contact with it'.

One can see the similarity between the two words. 'Force' is used in both definitions, but the adjectives used to define 'stress'; 'constraining' and 'impelling', convey a stronger feeling than the one used for 'pressure'; 'continuous'. More importantly, 'pressure' is force 'upon or against', while 'stress' carries with it the notion of 'force . . . between'. Etymologically, then, stress is not quite the same as pressure.

Engineers use another word for 'pressure' when talking about forces acting upon or against an object. Their word is 'load'. 'Loads', in engineering terms, produce stress and strain. But, as can be seen in Figure 2, that is not the end of the matter. Overload produces overstress. More load still can bring a piece of metal to a point where it begins to yield. Up to the yield-point a piece of metal will revert to its former dimensions when the load or overload is removed, but, when yielding sets in, it becomes impossible for metal to return to its original condition. Yielding causes irreversible strain. Continued overloading produces rupture and breakdown. Breakdown can result also from fatigue, a word frequently heard in connection with aircraft accidents. Fatigue is induced by frequent applications of load and overload. So much for the engineering approach. What about stress in relation to human beings?

One obvious point of difference is, that when used in relation to people, not all pressure, or load, produces stress. In fact, the opposite may be true. A person subject to no pressure at all may

What is Stress?

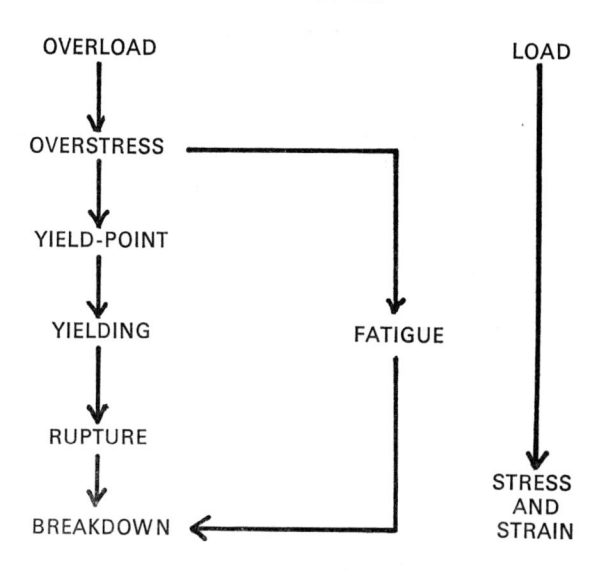

```
OVERLOAD                    LOAD
   │                         │
   ▼                         │
OVERSTRESS ─────────┐        │
   │                │        │
   ▼                │        │
YIELD-POINT         │        │
   │                │        │
   ▼                ▼        │
YIELDING         FATIGUE     │
   │                │        │
   ▼                │        ▼
RUPTURE             │     STRESS
   │                │      AND
   ▼                │     STRAIN
BREAKDOWN  ◄────────┘
```

Figure 2   Stress – in engineering terms

well begin to show signs of stress. Unemployment can have a very depressing effect on people who want to work. Under-employment, although not as demoralizing as being out of work, can lead to acute job dissatisfaction. A certain amount of pressure appears to be necessary if human beings are to develop and mature and make a creative contribution to society. People have a tremendous capacity for work, particularly creative work. A person can be under quite heavy pressure at work and still take on responsibilities in the community without showing stress signs. The problem for humans is not load, but overload; or no load.

The overload situation is the most common. The effect of pressure on a human being can best be described by thinking of a column of liquid in a tube. Figure 3 represents a normal, healthy person. Pressures are bearing down upon him, but his energy resources are such that his ability to cope (represented by the level of liquid) is well above his coping capacity, and nowhere near his point of breakdown. A human being's coping capacity corresponds to the yield-point in a rod or bar of metal, but it is infinitely more variable. While the level of pressure remains above a person's yield-point he remains mentally healthy, responds positively to challenges, enjoys life and develops as a normal person. The distance between a man or a woman's pressure level and their coping capacity or yield-point is dependent on two things; the amount of pressure being exerted and the position of the yield-point. The yield-point may

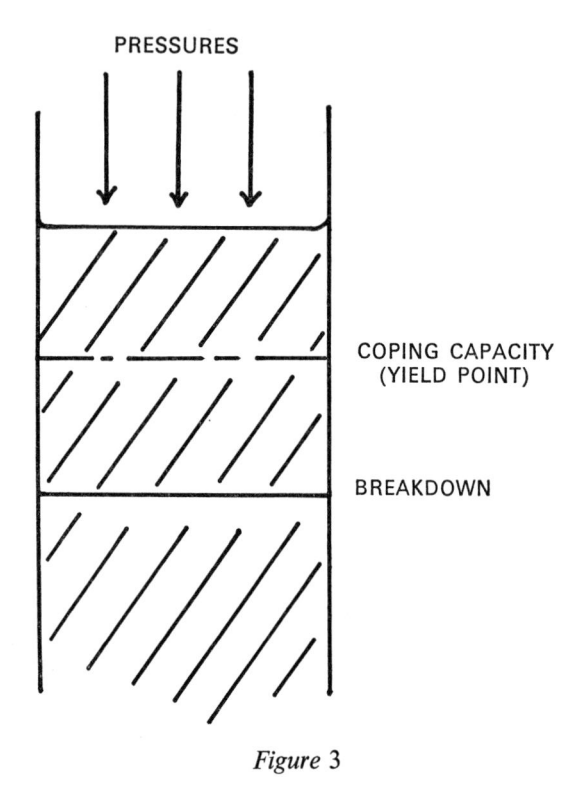

Figure 3

vary throughout the course of one day. Pressures may remain constant during a morning and an afternoon's work, but a worker may be able to achieve much more in one period than in the other. A woman in menstruation may find it much more difficult to be pleasant to everybody than at other times in the month. During menopause she may discover that she is no longer able to do the job she has done quite happily for the last twenty years. The problem is not so much increased load (to go back to engineering terminology) but reduced capacity to cope and this is caused by a rising yield-point. Figure 4 shows the effect of a rising yield-point. Resources are reduced to a minimum although the level of liquid in the tube remains the same.

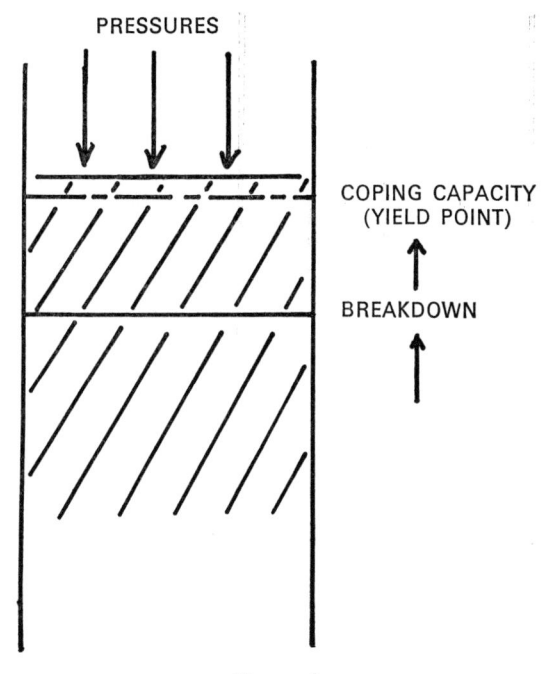

Figure 4

There are three things to be said at this point. One is that a person in this situation is still in a state of comparative ease. He has not yet gone beyond the point where dis-ease begins to show. The second point worth mentioning is that a rising yield-point may be quite undetectable. Unless a person, say, has been watching the number of hours he sleeps at night and making sure that he gets what, for him, is an adequate amount of rest, he may be completely oblivious to the fact that his reserves are low. Only when he is on the verge of making some irritable and uncharacteristic comment will he begin to be aware that he is not far away from a stress situation. The third point should now be obvious. In contrast to the stress engineers talk about, which is caused by external loading, human stress is caused by both external and internal forces. Stress signs begin to show when the level of pressure falls below the coping capacity or the human yield-point. This is illustrated at Figure 5. A person still has

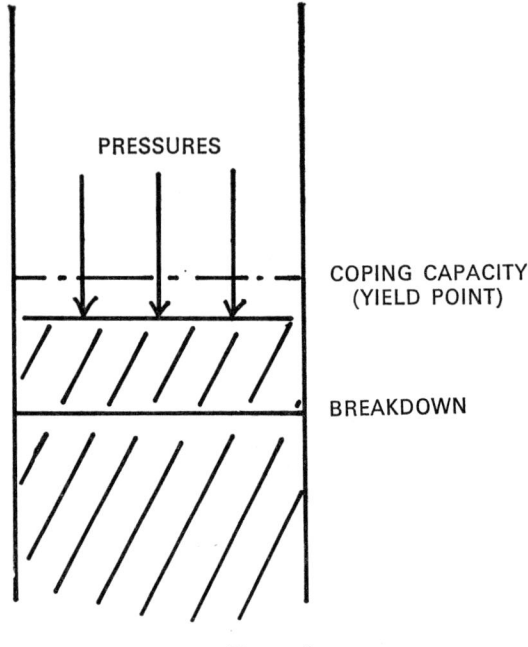

Figure 5

resources left, but they are the ones he would normally require to keep in a healthy state of mind. He has moved, if you like, from the black into the red; from a state of ease into a state of dis-ease. The interest he has to pay on what he borrows from his capital is measurable in stress symptoms. The more he draws, the deeper into trouble he gets and the nearer he approaches breakdown. He can do one of three things. He can either find a way of reducing his load, or, by some personal action, attempt to lower his yield-point, or he can ignore his developing symptoms and plunge onwards to danger.

Here, again, a contrast has to be made between human stress and the engineer's term. When a rod or a bar of metal has been

What is Stress?

loaded beyond its yield-point the consequences are irreversible. The metal is never quite the same again. Human beings are much more resilient. The fact that a man or woman is under stress does not mean that breakdown is inevitable, nor does it mean that irreversible damage has been done to the system. A person who has gone beyond his yield-point into a stress situation can pull back. He can regain a state of ease where he can cope positively with quite considerable amounts of pressure. Not all stress is damaging, but it is potentially damaging and the worse and more prolonged it is the greater are the chances that irreparable harm will be done. Figure 6 indicates that a breaking

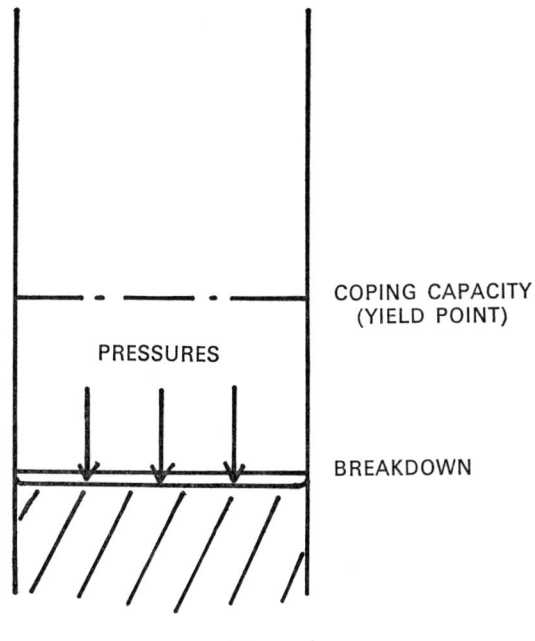

Figure 6

point can be reached when all but the emergency resources capable of maintaining minimum life-support systems are exhausted. A human being can recover even from this parlous state with care and expert treatment, but, if he has not destroyed part of himself in the process he may well find that his chances of promotion to greater responsibility are doomed.

Take Dick's case. Tension had been building up inside him for weeks. He never seemed able to get more than two-thirds the way down the pile of back-log on his desk. After a particularly hectic week a friend dropped him at the end of his road having given him a lift from work. Dick hadn't far to walk; about sixty yards. He almost reached his house. He collapsed on the pavement. Neighbours went for his wife. The doctor was telephoned. Dick looked dead. He almost was. The doctor examined him and ordered him to bed. His nervous system had given way under the pressure of work. The diagnosis was stress. Dick spent the next few weeks under heavy sedation. Slowly his energy came back. He eventually returned to work, still on tablets. His work was reorganized to take off some of the load. He survived. The experience taught him a lot. The day came when he was well enough to do without the pills. He looked as though he had recovered. About a year later he chose to be made redundant rather than take a job at a much lower level in the company. The remarkable thing was that he was able to live through the trauma of having to lose his job without suffering from a second breakdown. His friends at work probably helped him a lot. They encouraged him to look for alternative work. He had little difficulty in finding it; nearer home and at a higher salary.

Other people are less fortunate. A coronary thrombosis or cerebral haemorrhage can inflict irreparable damage. They may recover sufficiently to go back to work, but, without job redesign or the support of friends, stress quickly builds up again and they have to leave. Despite expert treatment in hospital, some never recover to do more than a light job. Others do not survive the ride in the ambulance.

MacNalty's *British Medical Dictionary* describes stress as, 'Any potentially damaging strain, force or agent which stimulates a physiological defense reaction and is capable under certain circumstances of producing pathological lesions.' This is almost an engineering definition. Dr. Joseph L. Kearns, a medical adviser to a large British company, writing in his book *Stress in Industry* (p. 28), takes a different line. 'Stress,' he says, 'is the internal condition of an individual' which is brought about by external stressors.

Apart from indicating a certain amount of confusion within the medical profession, neither of these definitions is satisfactory.

What is Stress?

Dr. Kearns is nearer the truth when he describes stress as 'an internal condition'. It is also true to say that stress is 'potentially damaging'. But, rather than being a 'force or agent', it is an omnibus word which covers a wide range of mental and physical disorders. The stress condition is recognizable by a variety of symptoms. These symptoms can be caused by internal as well as external forces. Not all forces or 'agents' produce stress. Stress only occurs when a person is 'loaded' beyond yield-point. The stress condition may last for a long time, particularly if there is a nagging worry in the back of a person's mind, or it may disappear in the course of a twenty-minute car ride from a stressed working environment to a relaxed and supportive domestic environment. Stress may range from the very slight, recognizable only by odd outbursts of irritability, to the very severe where a dozen or more signs might be identifiable. In the diagnosis and treatment of stress it is important to mark the progression of the condition. Like cancer, the earlier it can be caught the better are the chances of preventing a serious situation developing. This means that relatives, friends and workmates need to be alert to the signs of stress long before a problem develops which merits a visit to the factory doctor or general practitioner.

Hans Selye, a Canadian biochemist, describes three stages of stress: the Alarm Stage of shock and counter-shock; the Resistance Stage where defence measures are brought into action and the Exhaustion Stage which can lead, if the stress is persistent or very heavy, to physical and/or mental decline and death. It may be argued that stress does not always come as a result of sudden and unexpected and heavy loading. More than likely it will appear as a result of a slow and steady and imperceptible build-up; a problem that creeps up on a person almost without warning. Selye's Alarm Stage, for many, may well be non-existent.

A definition of stress may now be attempted.

Stress is a potentially damaging internal condition which can be recognized by a wide range of mental and physical disorders and brought on by internal or external forces. It can be very slight, ranging to very severe. It can be of short or longer duration and it appears when a person is loaded beyond his or her capacity to cope.

Chapter Four

The Stress Symptoms

The people in the packaging department worked well as a team. They made a significant contribution to the overall productivity of the firm. Invariably, they achieved their monthly targets and everyone was willing to work overtime to clear back log when, for one reason or another, the supply of parts was delayed. The high performance was due in no small measure to the supervisor; a hard working and conscientious person who took his work seriously and gained considerable satisfaction from being one of the most successful team leaders in the firm. He worked long hours and was a fine example to the rest. Very often he could be found, with his wife, enjoying a drink with people from his department in a pub after working hours. He was respected and liked.

It was difficult to say precisely when a stress situation began to develop in the department, but the workers became conscious, over a period, that their supervisor was beginning to behave rather oddly. He began to do things quite out of character. It was impossible for them to get him to talk, and, even though relationships were good, he was the supervisor. The workers watched him become more and more depressed. Their concern increased when he began to criticize them over quite trivial matters. If the girls were a few minutes late after going to the toilet he would become irritable and bad tempered. This was most unusual. There were days when they watched him at his desk, pencil in hand and documents before him but, obviously, unable to concentrate on his work. Performance, inevitably, fell off and the farther behind they got the worse the situation became. The men argued that it was management's responsibility to do something. The women said that it was his wife's duty to insist that a doctor be called in. The crisis came one afternoon just before tea-break. The supervisor collapsed with sharp pains across his chest and was rushed to hospital suffering from a coronary thrombosis. A hasty reorganization had to be made to keep the department running. It was some months before the supervisor returned to work.

It usually takes a situation like this to draw attention to the existence of stress at work, but the stress was evident long before the final tragedy. If the symptoms had been recognized and action taken sooner the hospitalization might have been avoided altogether. Problems could have been aired and resolved. Pressures could have been eased a little here and increased a bit there. Support could have been provided. Treatment could, perhaps, have been prescribed. The supervisor might have been alerted to what was happening to himself and taken steps to prevent a deterioration in health. Performance might well have been maintained through work sharing; perhaps, even, improved. Dislocation need never have happened. Industrial relations, instead of becoming soured, could have been kept at a high level. The cost of remedial action would have been a fraction of the cost eventually borne by the firm in lost production, sick pay and the wages of someone else to do the job, not to mention the worry and anxiety of a family at home and colleagues at work.

Stress is difficult, if not impossible, to hide. Some people, like Adam's secretary in Chapter One, will be able to tell on sight whether a person is under stress or not. For others, the stress signs will not be immediately obvious. But, as stress worsens, everyone will know. Work will slow down, memos will not be answered, people will become withdrawn, hesitant, indecisive and unreasonable. Casual absence may well increase and people may not only become more accident prone, but take longer to recover. Problems will be projected on to others and all personal responsibility for hold-ups disclaimed. The obvious could be strenuously denied. Attitudes might change quite fundamentally, and a normally placid person could become aggressive. These are some of the things that everyone sees. They are the external signs of an inward stress problem and, as such, need to be recognized as secondary symptoms. The primary symptoms are the ones which are much more personal and are directly linked with a person's inability to cope in a satisfactory, healthy and creative way with the pressures bearing down upon him. Into this category come symptoms such as depression, anxiety, irritability and a wide range of physical disorders which have roots in mental diseases.

Doctors group emotional disorders of this sort into three main sections; neuroses, psychoneuroses and psychoses.

A neurosis is a personality illness which can bring about a derangement of the mind or body. Neuroses are fairly common and do not necessarily lead to mental breakdown. A 'born worrier', for instance, can find himself, or herself, suffering from 'anxiety neurosis'. This may well be the wording on the medical certificate that eventually finds its way to the factory nurse. A person suffering from such an illness will be anxious, apprehensive, afraid and may be showing some physical signs, such as a skin rash or a recurring headache. The condition can be treated to relieve the anxiety, allay the fears and remove the physical disorders; at least, until pressure builds up again. Throughout all this, understanding, awareness and insight are retained by the patient. The loss of insight and awareness indicates a much more serious mental disorder. This is a psychosis. A depressive psychosis, for example, is an illness which plunges a person into a state of melancholia, depression and despondency. In this situation reasoning with a sufferer can have little or no effect; expert medical attention is required.

Psychoneurosis covers a group of mental disorders characterized by a faulty emotional response to pressure. This can show itself in a variety of ways. Anxiety state, hysteria and reactive depression are some examples. The information published by the Office of Health Economics in 1971 showed that between 1954 and 1968 the number of days lost from work through psychoneurosis and psychosis increased by 152 per cent for men and 302 per cent for women.

Doctors are by no means unanimous in their opinions about the relationship between stress and disease, but arguments have been advanced in medical textbooks to show the link between stress and a wide variety of physical disorders. Stress can cause over-eating, which, in turn, can produce obesity. Other addictions; to alcohol, smoking and drugs, can develop. A group of supervisors discussing the effects of stress agreed that it reduced their ability to have satisfactory sexual intercourse. Many medical practitioners believe that stress can be a factor in rheumatic disorders, rheumatoid arthritis, gout and allergic states. There seems to be wide agreement that blood pressure can be affected by stress, increasing the pumping action of the heart and the flow of blood through the arteries, capillaries and veins. It is felt that stress can aggravate heart abnormalities and help bring on thrombosis. It can produce hypertension.

The digestive system can be upset by stress. A person may suffer from loss of appetite or find difficulty in digesting certain foods. Long-term indigestion can bring on inflammation of the colon, known as ulcerative colitis, and peptic or stomach ulcers.

Recurring headaches can appear as a result of stress and attacks of migraine, a particularly debilitating illness which can include head pains, vomiting, flashes of light and a diminution of sight, may be worsened by stress. Other aches can occur in neck and jaw muscles.

Stress can affect sleep and long periods of tiredness can follow nights (or days) of shallow and disturbed rest. A person in this condition cannot give of his best at work.

Anxiety can be induced by stress. The medical dictionaries define it as an emotion condition in which feelings of fear, dread and mental agitation predominate. 'Situation anxiety' describes the sense of nervous apprehension which afflicts a person when starting a new job, or meeting a group of strangers, or when facing the threat of short-time working or redundancy

Depression has already been referred to. It is usually understood to be an attitude of unhappiness and hopelessness. Anxious, agitated depression is depression accompanied by anxiety and restlessness. Reactive depression may well follow a time of particularly heavy stress, say, through the loss of a member of the family after a long illness, or the loss of a job, or after months of inability to find suitable work.

Indications that a person is under stress can be observed in sudden outbursts of temper, irritability and inability to concentrate on what has to be done. A person who normally can be relied on to produce work on time, may begin to procrastinate under stress conditions. Tension can replace an easy and relaxed approach to situations and people. A person may become so stressed as to find it difficult to stop his work in order to relax. This may occur when a person has a very high commitment to the achievement of a task. In this case overwork becomes, not a cause of stress, but a symptom. Because it means the further expension of energy it also adds to stress. Some symptoms are more serious than others. Dread of going to work, lack of interest in work and fear of health breakdown come into this category. It is possible to reach a point when it becomes difficult for the cause to be separated from the effect; one symptom triggering off another. Gilbert's fear of health breakdown in Chapter One arose because of an ache in his head which, itself, was a symptom of a fairly serious stress condition.

In 1970 the International Committee on Occupational Mental Health organized a seminar on Stress in Industry in the London area. One thing to emerge from their discussions was a character by the name of Hector the Hedgehog whom they likened to a person reacting in a pricklish way to various stressors, while trying to walk and balance his way along a tightrope, carrying a load, part of which he may have chosen and part of which may have been thrust on him. They suggested that the reactions of a person who becomes anxious and afraid when only part way along his tightrope are rather like those of a hedgehog rolling up into a prickly ball, clutching his load tightly to his chest. The difficulties of trying to do anything to help the hedgehog can be considerable. Having got near enough one has then to persuade the animal to uncurl before normality can be achieved. So, with human beings. There is a tendency to curl up under stress; to hide problems; even to resist offers of help. In description of stress at work among supervisors, which is given later on in the book, mention is made of those who were identified as being under very severe stress. Although all needed medical help only just over 40 per cent had been to a doctor during the previous twelve months. Their condition was so bad that they could not have been unaware of the effect of pressures upon them, yet, for one reason or another, they chose to keep the problem to themselves.

In a stress situation a cause can lead to an effect which, itself, can become another cause. Stress can not only grow within a person, it can spread to others. If a company, for example, works towards a series of monthly targets the chances are that by the end of the third week, a stress situation is developing at management level because production is seen to be lagging behind schedule. Directives are issued which cause line management to apply pressure on those who are responsible to them. Particular pressure is applied to those in charge of areas where production is being held up. If parts are short, hasty telephone

The Stress Symptoms

calls are made to suppliers. Transport has to be organized to shift goods quickly from A to B. There is time only for a cursory inspection of those goods before they are whipped off to the problem area. By the middle of Week Four the pace has noticeably quickened. People hover, their appetite for parts apparently insatiable. Urgent meetings are called. Procedures are short-circuited. Overtime reaches the union limit and goes beyond after frantic calls to the District Office for a dispensation. With three days to go there is still a back-log. Panic sets in. Every stop is pulled out to meet the target. It is finally attained. The boss is happy. The chief accountant is happy. The production planners are happy. The customers are happy. But the producers are exhausted; particularly the supervisors upon whom the main burden for implementation of plans and directives falls. Week One of a new month comes with a sigh of relief and then it is Week Four and panic-stations again.

A stress count taken in Week One will be quite different from one taken in Week Four, particularly among those with slight to moderate stress. This will be due, almost entirely, to environmental conditions, but it does indicate a problem for those wanting to identify stress levels in an organization. The information one gains from an investigation, may, like a company balance sheet, only indicate the situation in that company on a particular day. At another time stress levels, like cash-flows, might be quite different and only by a comparison between sets of data can trends be identified. But, how can stress levels be identified? Is it possible when there are so many variables acting on one situation at any given time? This is a problem that has frustrated a detailed study of stress at work for a long time.

Chapter Five

STRESS LEVELS

The argument so far has been that humans are different from lumps of metal. Not all loads borne by people produce stress. In fact, stress is only produced when a man or woman is pushed to a point, called a coping capacity, or yield-point, when they can no longer respond to pressures in what could be called a normal, healthy way. Both pressures and yield-point will fluctuate during the course of a day, but a normal and healthy situation could be described as one where energy expended in work is replaced by a process of relaxation, recreation and sleep so that, at the start of a new day, the energy reserves are not less than what they were at the beginning of the previous day. This is assuming, of course, that the person has not started off with a stress condition.

It has been argued that a stress condition can be recognized by a wide range of mental and physical symptoms. By inviting a person to list his stress symptoms it ought to be possible to obtain a rough estimate of his stress problem. This will provide a snap-shot of his stress condition at a particular time. The picture may be a bit blurred and out of focus, first time, because a person may not be able, accurately, to identify his symptoms. But, as his understanding of what stress is increases, it ought to be possible to get a clearer image. By taking a number of readings over a period it ought to be possible to discover whether a situation is becoming more or less stressed. By examining each person, either in a company or in a particular group, the level of stress, at any point in time, can be determined for the company or group.

The assessment of a stress level depends on much more than a listing of symptoms. The symptoms, themselves, vary in importance. Some stress signs may appear because an overload of pressure at work or in the home aggravates an existing disorder. Indigestion for more than a week, blood pressure and heart trouble come into this category. In an assessment of stress levels such symptoms would rate lower than those more directly caused by overload, such as recurring headaches, depression or anxiety. There are other signs, mentioned already, such as fear of health breakdown or dread of going to work which would rate higher still.

The Primary symptoms, rather than the Secondary ones, are the signs which, if identified, help to determine just how much stress a person is under. The more common ones are as follows:

- Duodenal or stomach ulcers
- Migraine
- Skin rashes
- Blood pressure
- Heart trouble
- Aches in jaw and neck muscles
- Indigestion (for longer than a week)
- Loss of temper
- Overwork
- Coronary thrombosis
- Recurring headaches
- Sleeplessness
- Periods of depression
- Feeling of stress
- Irritability
- Anxiety
- Long periods of tiredness
- Tension
- Tendency to leave things until the last minute
- Dread of going to work
- Lack of interest in work
- Fear of health breakdown

This is by no means an exhaustive list, but a rough idea of the level of stress in a person can be gained simply by asking a person to indicate which factor they can identify in themselves in a particular location at a particular time. Perhaps, a rough idea of the level of stress in a person at a particular time is all one is ever likely to obtain considering the many variables at work in any situation. But a series of 'stress temperatures' or 'stress photographs' taken at periods of, say, three or four months, could provide sufficient evidence to forestall a mental or physical breakdown. An increasing stress level would indicate that something, somewhere, was seriously wrong.

How is the stress level obtained? In the research that was done among supervisors; and, since, among various other groups of people, Duodenal or stomach ulcers down to Coronary thrombosis, scored 1; Recurring headaches to Tendency to leave things until the last minute, scored 2 and Dread of going to work, Lack of interest in work and Fear of health breakdown, all scored 3.

A person identifying Aches in jaw and neck muscles, Periods of depression, Irritability, Anxiety, Tendency to leave things until the last minute and Lack of interest in work, would have a total score of 12.

An investigation into the stress levels of a group of people could produce totals ranging from zero to over 20. Scores of 25 and 26 are not uncommon, but it is unlikely anyone would accumulate a maximum 37. A score of zero to 2 could indicate no stress, or very slight stress. A score of 3 to 6 would show slight stress, and, one of 7 to 12, moderate stress. A person with a count of 13 to 17 would be under severe stress and a score of 18 or over would indicate very severe stress. The person with a score of 12 would, therefore, come in at the top end of the moderate stress group and might be judged to be in need of help of some kind. His pattern of stress, that is, the type of symptoms being shown, would be the determining factor. A person with a very high score would be showing both mental and physical symptoms and would need to be advised to consult a doctor for some expert counselling and treatment. Figure 7 shows the list of symptoms together with scores and gradings.

An organization wanting to assess stress levels needs to remember that data will vary according to personality, occupation, environment and time. The best time to do a study might well be the most inconvenient time when pressures are great. If a firm worked a system in which pressures built up towards month end, it would be interesting to compare data collected in Week One with that collected in Week Four. Over a longer period it would be important to compare information from a series of Week Fours. This latter data would be the most useful in determining whether or not occupational health was improving or getting worse. When a person or a group of people is being presented with a list of symptoms and is asked to indicate which they can recognize in themselves they need to be clear that they are being asked to state what they are aware of in a particular situation at a particular time. Information collected over a short period will

Symptoms	Score	Range	Grade
Duodenal or stomach ulcers Migraine Skin rashes Blood pressure Heart trouble Aches in jaw and neck muscles Indigestion (for longer than a week) Loss of temper Overwork Coronary thrombosis	Score 1	0–2	*No or very slight stress*
		3–6	*Slight stress*
Recurring headaches Sleeplessness Periods of depression Feeling of stress Irritability Anxiety Long periods of tiredness Tension Tendency to leave things until the last minute	Score 2	7–12	*Moderate stress*
		13–17	*Severe stress*
		18 and over	*Very severe stress (requiring medical treatment)*
Dread of going to work Lack of interest in work Fear of health breakdown	Score 3		

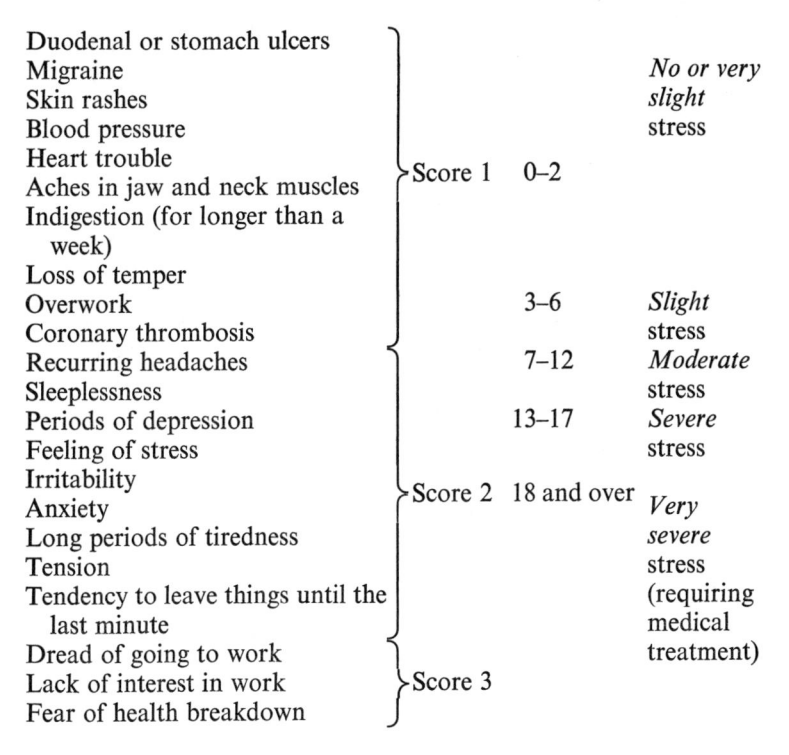

Figure 7 Symptoms, scores and grades

give a sharper picture of what is happening in an organization than data which takes weeks to gather. Stress levels are easy to identify, given how to score and grade the symptoms. The difficulties of an exercise of this sort lie, not in working out the sums, but in getting people to co-operate and, either, in distributing forms and instructions to wherever people are and collecting them again, or, in bringing those to be assessed to some central point in order to obtain the necessary information there. A sample form which would enable a researcher to work out levels of stress and give him, in addition, some indication of areas, within a working situation, which could be contributing to a stress problems, is shown at Figure 8.

Exercise
1. Look at the list of symptoms, scores and grades in Figure 7.
2. Tick off the symptoms which you feel you are suffering from. (*N.B.* This can reflect how you are feeling at the moment or you may wish to think yourself back into a recent working situation.)
3. Add up your score.
4. Work out your stress grading.
5. Make a plan to repeat the exercise in a week or so's time and compare results.
6. Discuss your findings with someone else.
7. If you feel your stress count is too high, take some positive action to lower it. (*N.B.* Simply talking over your problem may ease tension.)

Score: *Grade:*

1. NAME ....
2. AGE ....years
3. TITLE OF YOUR JOB
   ....
4. NO. OF YEARS IN PRESENT JOB ....
5. MAIN RESPONSIBILITIES
   ....
   ....
6. MOST TIME-CONSUMING TASKS
   ....
   ....
7. MAJOR WORK PROBLEMS
   ....
   ....
8. ARE YOU AT PRESENT UNDERGOING TREATMENT FROM YOUR DOCTOR?
   Yes/No
9. IF YOU THINK YOU MAY BE UNDER SOME STRESS UNDERLINE WHICH OF THE FOLLOWING YOU THINK IS THE MAIN CONTRIBUTORY FACTOR
   – problems at home
   – problems connected with work
   – your own personality
   – other factors
10. DATE WHEN FORM COMPLETED ......19..
11. LOCATION ....

Tick if you have any of the following:

Duodenal or stomach ulcers

Migraine

Skin rashes

Blood pressure

Heart trouble

Aches in jaw and neck muscles

Indigestion for longer than a week

Loss of temper

Overwork

Coronary thrombosis

Recurring headaches

Sleeplessness

Periods of depression

Feeling of stress

Irritability

Anxiety

Long periods of tiredness

Tension

Tendency to leave things until the last minute

Dread of going to work

Lack of interest in work

Fear of health breakdown

Figure 8 Stress Analysis form

Chapter Six

STRESS PATTERNS

Information obtained from a Stress Analysis form (see Figure 8) will provide not only a stress level for an individual person or a group of people in a particular occupation or a whole organization, it will also reveal stress patterns. As research develops in this field it may be possible, in time, to avoid the worst problems of mental ill-health by taking preventive action to overcome the symptoms commonly associated with specific groups or occupations.

At Allen's and Brown's, the two companies involved in the research into stress at work among supervisors, more than two-thirds of the men and women who took part showed signs of stress.

The first company, Allen's, was the smaller of the two, employing between five and six hundred people. A third of the production supervisors there showed no or very slight stress. Another third had slight stress, 20 per cent were under moderate stress and 6·67 per cent showed severe and very severe stress levels respectively. Their leading symptoms were: Loss of temper (40 per cent), Tension (33 per cent), Overwork (33 per cent), Long periods of tiredness (27 per cent), Irritability (20 per cent), Anxiety (20 per cent), Feeling of stress (20 per cent) and Sleeplessness (20 per cent).

At Brown's, a firm employing over two thousand people in a couple of highly mechanized and partially automated plants, stress levels among the production supervisors were much higher. Of these 39·6 per cent said they were not under stress, 18·9 per cent were under slight stress and 22·6 per cent had moderate stress. Also 15·1 per cent showed severe stress and 3·8 per cent very severe stress. Their leading symptoms were: Tension (43 per cent) Irritability (41 per cent), Feeling of stress (40 per cent), Overwork (38 per cent), Loss of temper (36 per cent), Long periods of tiredness (26 per cent), Anxiety (21 per cent) and Tendency to leave things until the last minute (19 per cent).

Stress Patterns

Apart from Sleeplessness and Tendency to leave things until the last minute the two stress patterns were remarkably similar. Tension and Overwork were high in both groups.

The supervisors not directly concerned with production were also studied in the two companies. At Allen's the non-production group had the highest average stress count. Although 30 per cent showed little or no stress, 20 per cent had slight stress, 40 per cent moderate stress and 10 per cent very severe stress. Their stress pattern was as follows: Irritability (60 per cent), Depression (40 per cent), Sleeplessness (40 per cent), Tension (40 per cent), Loss of temper (40 per cent), Overwork (40 per cent), Tendency to leave things until the last minute (30 per cent) and Feeling of stress (30 per cent).

Brown's non-production supervisors had the smallest group showing little or no stress – 27·6 per cent; 31 per cent had slight stress, 24·1 per cent moderate stress, 6·9 per cent severe stress and 10·4 per cent very severe stress. As a group they had the second highest stress count; higher than both production groups. Their stress pattern read: Irritability (41 per cent), Depression (35 per cent), Tension (35 per cent), Tendency to leave things until the last minute (35 per cent), Loss of temper (31 per cent), Anxiety (31 per cent) and Feeling of stress (28 per cent). Again, there were marked similarities between both non-production groups, with Irritability, Depression and Tension high in the lists.

The similarity of stress pattern between both production groups and both non-production groups was one interesting factor to emerge. The lower level of stress among production groups compared to their respective non-production colleagues was another and the high incidence of Depression among the non-production supervisors was the third notable factor.

The complete picture of the incidence of stress signs at the two firms is given at Figure 9. In order to give a true comparison between production and non-production groups at Allen's and Brown's the numbers in columns 2 and 4 have been multiplied by 1½ and 2 respectively.

It will be seen from Figure 9 that all four groups were remarkably free from blood pressure and heart disease problems. Only one person was shown to be suffering from coronary thrombosis. Among the production supervisors 13 per cent at

	Allen's		Brown's	
Stress Symptom	Column 1 Production Supervisor	Column 2 Non-Production Supervisor	Column 3 Production Supervisor	Column 4 Non-Production Supervisor
Duodenal or stomach ulcers	1	3	1	2
Migraine	—	1·5	6	2
Skin rashes	—	1·5	4	2
Blood pressure	—	—	—	—
Heart trouble	—	—	1	—
Aches in jaw and neck muscles	1	—	3	6
Indigestion for longer than a week	1	1·5	5	2
Loss of temper	6	6	19	18
Overwork	5	6	20	14
Coronary thrombosis	—	—	1	—
Recurring headaches	1	3	3	8
Sleeplessness	3	6	2	12
Periods of depression	1	6	9	20
Feeling of stress	3	4·5	21	16
Irritability	3	9	22	24
Anxiety	3	1·5	11	18
Long periods of tiredness	4	3	14	14
Tension	5	6	23	20
Tendency to leave things until the last minute	—	4·5	10	20
Dread of going to work	2	—	2	4
Lack of interest in work	2	1·5	7	6
Fear of health breakdown	2	3	5	—

Figure 9 Incidence of Stress at Allen's and Brown's – Comparative Figures

Allen's and 4 per cent at Brown's dreaded going to work. Another 13 per cent at both firms showed a lack of interest in work and 13 per cent at Allen's and 10 per cent at Brown's feared a health breakdown. No one among the non-production people at Allen's dreaded going to work, though 7 per cent at Brown's showed evidence of this problem. At both companies 10 per cent lacked interest in work and 20 per cent of the non-production supervisors at Allen's were afraid of a breakdown in health.

Figure 9 also shows the dominance of the mental over the physical symptoms. In a stress situation information of this nature is essential if the problem is to be properly evaluated and plans laid to resolve it.

Research among a group of student teachers a week before second-year teaching practice revealed 38 per cent under slight stress, 23 per cent under moderate stress, 31 per cent under severe stress and 8 per cent under very severe stress. Their stress pattern was: Irritability (62 per cent), Depression (54 per cent), Tendency to leave things until the last minute (54 per cent), Tension (46 per cent), Anxiety (38 per cent), Dread of going to work (31 per cent). Apart from one twenty-year-old who ran up a total score of 22 there were few signs of the physical symptoms of stress. No one declared a lack of interest in work.

Among a group of parsons on a retraining course 40 per cent were under slight stress, 45 per cent under moderate stress, 10 per cent under severe stress and 5 per cent under very severe stress. Their leading stress symptoms were: Loss of temper (65 per cent), Irritability (65 per cent), Overwork (60 per cent), Tendency to leave things until the last minute (60 per cent), Tension (30 per cent) and Long periods of tiredness (30 per cent).

A group of retired men showed a remarkable number under little or no stress – 48 per cent; 33 per cent were under slight stress, 5 per cent under moderate stress and 14 per cent under severe stress. Their stress pattern showed, as one might have expected, a higher incidence of the physical symptoms. Their leading signs were: Tendency to leave things until the last minute (33 per cent), Anxiety (29 per cent), Heart trouble (29 per cent), Fear of health breakdown (29 per cent), Loss of temper (19 per cent), Irritability (19 per cent), Sleeplessness (19 per cent), Periods of depression (19 per cent).

An analysis of stress symptoms is important not just to identify the leading signs, which, for supervisors, appear to be Irritability, Tension, Depression and Overwork, but to show up the less common, but, to the person concerned, significant symptoms. Study among a group of potential supervisors revealed five sufferers from migraine. Another study showed a comparatively high degree of lack of interest in work among a group of people whom one normally would not expect to show this sign.

The identification of stress levels and the discovery of stress patterns helps organizations to determine where the problems are. It gives them a basis on which to decide whether action is required or not; whether to launch into an overall programme or to concentrate activity in one or two areas. A series of studies helps to identify trends. There is no reason why this should not be done quickly and easily. But, it is one thing to persuade the boss that money should be spent on overcoming stress. It is much more difficult to decide Why, Where and How.

Chapter Seven

STRESS AT WORK AND IN THE COMMUNITY

It is the belief of some managers that a degree of stress is necessary within the working environment in order to get the best out of people. A degree of stress may be inevitable within the working environment but this is very different from saying that it is necessary. People who argue for the latter point of view probably are guilty of confusing pressure and stress. There is no doubt at all that pressure is necessary if maximum efficiency and productivity are to be achieved. Pressure, up to a point, can have a very positive effect. But stress is wholly negative. A person under stress is a person who is already showing signs of reaction to pressure; pressure that is being applied either by himself or from some outside source. The more the stress, the more the inefficiency. The primary symptoms, which are helpful in determining stress levels, lead to the secondary symptoms which create inter-personal and organizational problems. The former may be felt by the individual human being. The latter can quickly become clear to a wide range of other people. Few companies can afford the luxury of the kind of secondary stress symptoms listed in Chapter Four.

It is the aim of this book to underline the significance of the stress problem. It is also the aim of this book to point to the need for something to be done about stress within the working environment.

The twenty-three million or so people who are registered either as employed or unemployed in Britain are also subjects of government in a constantly changing industrial and economic environment and participants in a web of family, personal and community relationships of one kind or another. Society being what it is, it is just not possible to isolate one area from another.

Non-work factors influence industry and industry influences other sectors. The growth of the north-east of England from the middle of the nineteenth century onwards followed the exploitation of coal, iron and chemical resources and the construction of freight carrying and public railways. The closure of uneconomic pits in the 1950s and 1960s ripped the heart out of many Durham mining communities. Life changed dramatically for men who, for the first time in generations, had either to go on the dole or travel miles to find alternative work. Everyone was affected. The visible scars of once thriving and now derelict industrial communities are still to be seen as are the more hopeful signs of new towns and new industries. The British character, such as it is, owes a great deal to non-industrial factors, but there can be no doubt that community development and decline are closely related to industrial and economic fluctuations.

In 1800 the entire population of the northern towns of Darlington, Stockton, Hartlepool and Yarm numbered little more than 10,000. Middlesbrough did not exist. Twenty-five people lived in the area it now occupies, scratching a living from the land. Then, in 1825, came the first public railway in the world, running from Witton Park, Coundon and Haggerleazes in County Durham for twenty-six-and-three-quarter miles via Darlington to Stockton, lower down the River Tees, with a branch line to Yarm. Money was invested in the mines and coal exports rose to over one-and-a-half million tons by 1840. In 1850, when the population of Middlesbrough was barely 7,000, the main basic iron ore seam was discovered in the Cleveland Hills near by. By 1870 sixty-seven blast furnaces were producing 916,970 tons of pig iron. Middlesbrough's population was 39,000.

The impact of technical change was vividly demonstrated in the transition from iron making to steel. Henry Bessemer perfected his process for the manufacture of steel in large quantities using acidic ore in 1856. Sheffield was the first British centre of the new industry. Partly because the ore in the Cleveland Hills was unsuitable, being of the basic kind, the north-east lagged behind the Midlands in steel making. A Bessemer plant opened at Spennymoor in 1861, using imported ore. As late as 1872 no steel of any kind was made in the Middlesbrough area. Iron was supreme in the boom years of the late 1860s and early 1870s. The first Bessemer plant was built at Eston, near Middlesbrough, in 1876. Dividends were dropping and many iron firms were going into liquidation. The year 1879 saw heavy depression and unemployment at a time when Middlesbrough's population was over 50,000. That year, a process for making steel from local basic ore was demonstrated at the Bolckow and Vaughan works in the town. This open hearth process required an enormous plant. The increasing size of plant created new patterns of relationships at work. The next twenty years saw the development of the steel industry and the rapid decline of iron. Another 40,000 people were added to Middlesbrough's population, which, by 1901, reached 91,302. Managers took the place of employers who receded from the workplace. Terms of work were set increasingly by bargaining between trade unions and employers. The captains of industry, the entrepreneurs of the first industrial revolution, moved out of town to large houses in the country. This curtailed their contribution to life in the community outside the factory. They became less familiar with the problems of the area. Commercial development made Middlesbrough more dependent on financial initiatives taken elsewhere. The local economy, towards the end of the century, was drawn more and more into the national economy. By 1900 the majority of working men in this area of the north-east lived on the borderline between want and poverty. Social insecurity was at the heart of the industrial and urban system.

The town developers, such as they were, grouped workers and their families close to places of employment in rows of cheap, easily constructed and accessible terraced houses. The close relationships created by this kind of community has been a significant factor in northern working-class areas. But another revolution, the rapid decline of traditional industries such as mining, heavy engineering, railway locomotive manufacture and agriculture, has been powerful enough throughout the 1950s, 1960s and 1970s to transform community life, to break close kinship ties and brutalize many warm, friendly, caring and creative towns and villages.

A concrete sprawl of flats and maisonettes; limited to a few storeys in height because of the possibilities of mining subsidence, stands on the site of the old Bessemer plant at Spennymoore. A few miles away, across the Durham countryside, Witton Park is half derelict. The old Iron Masters district of Middlesbrough, once a centre of thriving activity, is being cleared for future development. The area is so heavily polluted atmospherically that it is unlikely to be used for housing schemes.

Outdated industrial plant still exists, breeding a reluctance to change. How sharply it contrasts with the new, capital intensive structures, where an investment of a million pounds creates a handful of jobs. The transition from one type of work to another creates many employment problems. The introduction of light industry draws women to work, dislocating the traditional pattern of north-east family life. The rapid growth of science-based industry and professional and administrative jobs calls for a radical improvement in higher educational opportunities. Young people are driven away from home in their search for suitable work. It isn't just industry that is producing changed attitudes and characters, but there can be no doubt that it is the dominant force shaping future patterns of society for better or for worse.

Stresses in communities struggling with the disorderliness of growth and the dislocation of change are likely to be high. Because man is at one and the same time a worker, a subject of government and a participator in a web of family, personal and community relationships, what happens in the community must have an influence on what happens at work. Similarly, what happens at work must have some impact on what happens elsewhere. The ideal is to have a flourishing industry, within which man has opportunity to grow and develop, and a flourishing community where he and others can advance educationally, culturally, spiritually, and socially, aided by adequate facilities and community services. But the reality is often far from the ideal.

Karl Marx and Friedrich Engels, writing in the mid-nineteenth century, were among the first to point to the alienating effect of work on man. Marx produced his thoughts on Alienated Labour in an unfinished manuscript in 1844. Alienation he regarded as a fact even in those early days. Looking at the relationship of the worker to the objects of his production he argued that the increasing value of the world of things proceeds in direct proportion to the devaluation of the world of men. Marx outlined four areas of alienation: estrangement between the worker and the object he produces; estrangement, in the act of production, of the worker from himself; estrangement of man from nature and estrangement of man from man, which, because of the practical relationships existing between men, leads them to regard one another as alien, hostile, powerful and independent. 'It is true,' said Marx, 'that labour produces for the rich wondderful things – but for the worker it produces privation. It produces palaces – but for the worker, hovels. It produces beauty – but for the worker, deformity. It replaces labour by machines – but some of the workers it throws back to a barbarous type of labour, and the other workers it turns into machines. It produces intelligence – but for the worker idiocy, cretinism.'

Engels, with Lancashire textile workers in mind, said, 'Nothing is more terrible than being constrained to do some one thing every day from morning until night against one's will. And the more a man the worker feels himself, the more hateful must his work be to him, because he feels the constraint, the aimlessness of it for himself. Why does he work? For love of work? From a natural impulse? Not at all. He works for money, for a thing which has nothing whatsoever to do with the work itself . . . The division of labour has multiplied the brutalising influences of forced work. In most branches the worker's activity is reduced to some paltry, purely mechanical manipulation, repeated minute after minute, unchanged year after year.' (*The Condition of the Working Class in England in 1844.*)

Engels was very pessimistic about the effect of continued technical change. He felt that work would become so meaningless and the rewards would be so limited for the working classes that they would revolt. Both Engels and Marx saw the link between what a man did at work and what he did afterwards. The former was particularly aghast at the intemperance and sexual licence exhibited by the working class during their leisure hours. 'This,' he argues, 'follows with relentless logic, with inevitable necessity, out of the position of a class left to itself, with no means of making fitting use of its freedom.'

Eric Fromm, writing a hundred years later, asked, in his book, *The Sane Society*, 'Is man, during the next few hundred years, to continue to spend most of his energy on meaningless work, waiting for the time when work will hardly require any expenditure of energy? What will become of him in the meantime? Will he not become more and more alienated, and this just as much in his leisure hours as in his working time?'

The nature of a man's work, both what he does and how he does it, and the complex relationships that surround him at work, have a marked effect upon him, not only at work but at home and in his leisure as well. Not every man is diminished by work, but some are, and the stresses so created have a wide rather than a narrow influence.

In the mid-1960s James Lawson worked as a cranedriver at Joseph Henshaw's, a heavy engineering firm manufacturing large castings for the steel and shipping industry. He was thirty-six years of age, married, and had three children, all boys. The eldest was eight years old. James, and his wife, Margaret, lived in a small, two-up-and-two-down terraced house built in 1890; one of hundreds of workers' dwellings surrounding a large and, now, half-derelict industrial site on the eastern side of the town.

Henshaw's was convenient; just five minutes' walk away from home. James had been there nearly nine years. He liked his job and was good at it; controlling the lighter loads just as well as the heavy sixty-ton ones. The relationship he had with the men on the shop floor was good. It was close. It had to be. Their lives were often in his hands as he moved castings from one end of the shop to the other. They worked very much as a team. From his cab James could see everything going on, right over three shops.

The problem at Henshaw's was the money. Working a basic $42\frac{1}{2}$ hour week barely earned him enough to keep going. He had to work overtime and weekends to boost his wage. He needed all the money he could get, especially as he and Margaret wanted to buy the house they were living in. An £850 mortgage and ever increasing interest rates was a burden for a man drawing a cranedriver's wage.

James decided to change jobs. The prospect of earning more elsewhere was the major factor, but James was also conscious that work was less plentiful at Henshaw's. Less and less overtime was being worked and rumours of impending closure were in the air. He could either wait and collect a lump sum in redundancy money or make a move.

The week after his thirty-seventh birthday James wrote off for a job as a semi-skilled machine operator at a new company in the town. At his interview he was offered employment at £4 a week more than what Henshaw's were paying and only for a

40-hour week. Overtime prospects were good. James was pleased. He handed in his notice and, at the end of the week, gave up his cranedriving job. Both he and Margaret felt that he had done the right thing.

James started his new job at 8 a.m. the following Monday. He was taken to an office where he signed a contract of employment and received a copy of the firm's Labour Agreement. He was then introduced to a supervisor and led off, along with four others, along a corridor, through the canteen, and into the machine shop. He couldn't help but compare it with Henshaw's. It was low roofed, packed with machines and lit by artificial light. So far as James could see there were no over-head cranes. Nor were there any windows. Men were working away at machines set out in long lines. Metal baskets full of machined parts were being pushed along rollers from one man to another.

James was taken to the far end of the shop. The supervisor pointed out a group of ten machines, each doing a simple operation on a small metal casting about five inches long called a rocker lever. The process was explained and James was shown how to operate one of the machines.

Although he had never seen a machine quite like it before, he found the task quite simple. All he had to do was to pick up a casting with one hand, remove a finished one with the other, locate the new casting in its proper place on the machine and press a button to his right. Machined castings were packed side by side in a metal basket and pushed along the rollers to the man at the next machine. It took James about half-an-hour to get into the rhythm of work.

The morning passed quite quickly and it was lunch time before James had a chance to talk to some of the other men in the section. He found that all of them had come from very different backgrounds; some from the mines, others from long-distance lorry driving and some from railway workshops. Quite a lot had been made redundant. He enjoyed his canteen meal.

At the end of the day he felt he had done pretty well, but he was a bit staggered when his supervisor told him that he was expected to machine far more castings in a normal, working day.

Over the first few weeks James's interest in the job began to wane. Compared to his previous job, this one carried little or no responsibility. There was no question of other people's lives being at risk. Little could go wrong. The machine did the work. James had to watch his fingers did not get scratched or trapped. The machine oil was a nuisance, soaking his overall now and then, but that was all. Sometimes the machine stopped and James learned from the others where to hit it with the hammer to get it going again. When this failed he reported it to the supervisor, who called in a setter, who got it going again. While this was happening James was put on another machine.

In the first twelve months James worked on all ten machines in the section. Each one was very much like the other. Once the rhythm of work had been mastered there were few difficulties. During the year James worked out that he must have handled not hundreds, but thousands and thousands of castings. He began to wonder where they all went to. Could there be a ship somewhere dumping them into the sea?

He persevered. There was little alternative. The mortgage was being paid off. Margaret was expecting again. After a long battle between the union and the management everyone in the section got a £2 per week rise. At least, James thought, that was some compensation for how he felt about work. But he knew it wasn't adequate. It didn't help him to feel more of a man and less of an extension to the machines. It did little to ease the dread of going to work that he began to get in the mornings. It didn't make him more of a thinking person as he was moved from machine to machine.

James saw an Inspector's job advertised on the work's noticeboard. He did not know how to use the equipment he saw other inspector's using, but he applied for the vacancy. He wasn't hopeful at all. He had had only a secondary modern school education. He wasn't apprenticed trained. A fortnight went by. He heard nothing. Increasingly sick of his work he wondered if night shift would be any better. At least the longer weekends would give him more time to forget about rocker-levers.

James started to work nights; four ten-hour shifts from Monday to Thursday, 9.30 p.m. to 8 o'clock in the morning. There was less supervision at night and the extra shift-premium to add to his basic wage. He liked the chance to get on with his job without interruption. He was able to work steadily through his regular quota of castings, making up a bit of time here and there for an extended smoke and a chat. But, in other ways, James found nights worse than days. Unless something went wrong with the machine he got stuck on one machine for the whole of the ten hours. His problems grew rather than lessened.

After six months, sometimes on nights, sometimes on days, James's frustrations began to show at home in quarrels and bickerings over little things. Normally quiet and good natured, he found himself increasingly irritated by the children. There were tensions, tears, upsets, shoutings and slammed doors. Even at the club, James found it difficult to relax. After a drink or two he wanted to go home. Invariably, Margaret, out of the house for a few hours, wanted to stay. Trouble flared up again.

James was sick of rocker-levers, sick of work, sick of feeling the way he did. He had never earned so much nor felt so miserable.

The climax came one night just before Christmas. Foolishly, James agreed to go with a mate to pick up some scrap lying about on a disused factory site. The prospect of a bit of excitement to break the monotony of work lured him rather than the possibility of earning a few extra pounds. They were caught in the act and James spent the night in a cell at the local police station. He was terrified of what might happen. Margaret, who came to visit him the next day, was heart-broken.

The weekend James spent, locked up, was the most humiliating in his life. He was scared stiff of being sent to prison. At the Magistrate's Court on the Monday morning he got away with a fine.

Nobody said a thing at work the next day, but James knew he had reached a turning point. He either had to get another job elsewhere in the firm or hand in his notice.

The name is fictitious but the story is true. James's life is now being lived out in a much more varied and challenging job and in happier and vastly healthier circumstances both for him and his growing family. His experience is not untypical. There are many thousands of men feeling the same kind of alienation and showing the same stress signs without really being able to understand why such problems should arise and how they can be sorted out. It could be argued that his problems were entirely of his own making; that he should have recognized that things were going wrong and got out before others became involved.

But many people lack both the freedom and the courage to do that. Neither industry nor society can abdicate its responsibility to identify where the stress-producing areas are. It is not enough to push the problem back on to the individual human being and, at the same time, organize work in such a way that men have to spend long hours in unchallenging and almost meaningless activity. Nor is it enough to imagine that more money for less work or a more creative use of leisure will be sufficient to compensate for the ill-health induced by such a working environment. In addition to finding a way to share wealth more justly and fairly among the world's people and in addition to creating more leisure and the facilities and education to enable the world's people to make a creative use of it, there has to be a willingness, both on the part of trade unions and management, to bring about radical changes in the stress-inducing areas of work. To alter an old saying slightly. 'Of what benefit is it to a man to gain the whole world and lose his health and well-being in the process?'

Chapter Eight

STRESS AND THE SUPERVISOR

The history of the iron and steel industry shows that the development of large-sized plants removed the employer from day-to-day contact with the worker and created the need for the appointment of the professional manager. As industrial organizations developed, the manager came to rely heavily on his foremen; authoritative figures in the first half of the twentieth century, with responsibilities to implement orders from above, to control and supervise work in hand and with power to fire as well as hire as many employees as the firm thought fit. The foreman was a formidable figure; bowler-hatted and commanding, sturdy, white-collared, upstanding and proud. Nepotism, the undue preferment of sons, nephews and other relatives, spoiled his chances of promotion, but his job was fairly secure. He could look forward to a gold watch after twenty-five years' service and a small pension, perhaps, when he retired. His status, power and authority placed him firmly in the ranks of management. The short line of command to the top meant that his word carried weight.

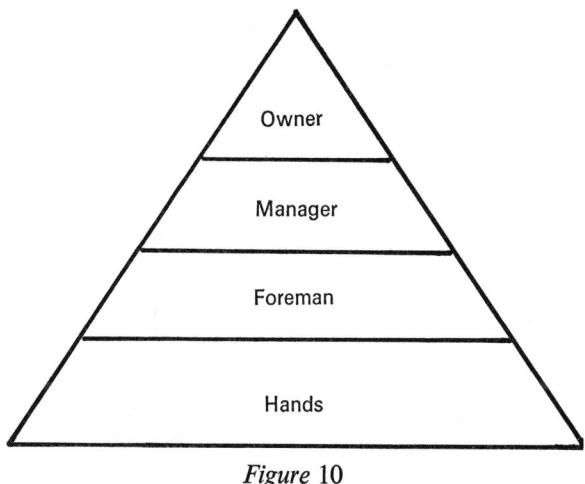

Figure 10

Organizations, particularly family businesses, were not unlike the pyramid structure shown in Figure 10. Owner–manager–foremen–hands was a fairly straightforward set-up. People knew their place. Communications came down from above. Loyalty and obedience to the firm were expected. Changes were few.

T. Burns and G. M. Stalker describe this rather static and mechanistic organization in their book, *The Management of Innovation*, published by Tavistock Publications Ltd. in 1961. They contrast it with the more flexible and organic organizations which have grown up in recent years as a result of industrial, economic, commercial and technical change.

The modern foreman or supervisor still retains his responsibilities for the implementation of plans. He is still at the point of interaction between management and the 'hands', but, in almost every other respect, his situation has radically changed.

The pyramid is no longer a meaningful diagram to illustrate the present position of many supervisors. Figure 11 gives a

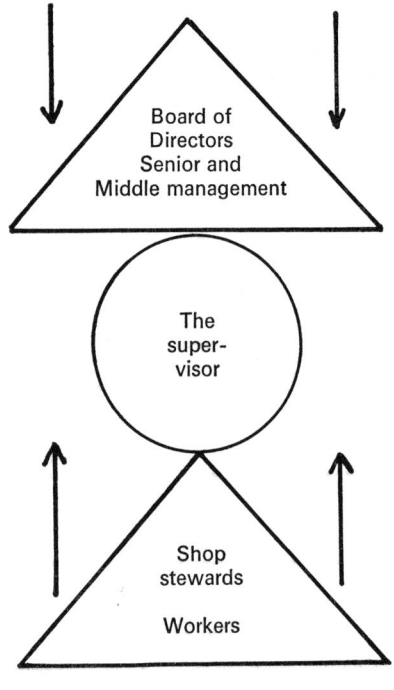

Figure 11

better indication of the situation in which many men and women find themselves. An era of merger, take-over, rationalization, nationalization, multi-nationals and conglomerates has pushed ownership even farther from the production area. Responsibility for setting profit margins and production targets may rest with a board of directors many thousands of miles away from where the supervisor is employed. Lines of communication have not only lengthened geographically, they have lengthened and broadened functionally as well. The increasing size and complexity of organizations has meant the introduction of additional levels of management. Many more people have to be consulted now before decisions can be made. All kinds of staff personnel have been taken on board ship in order to help service those with a direct responsibility for producing the goods. The managers of subsidiary companies are often employees rather than employers. They may have retained responsibility but much of their authority has been taken from them. The growth of management unions for protection purposes is one indication of this trend. This has meant a subsequent loss of authority for the supervisor. Decisions about important matters have now to be taken at much higher levels in the organizational network.

The creation of an organizational network, and it is a network rather than a ladder, has opened up greater prospects for advancement for the supervisor, provided, of course, he has the ability and the necessary academic and professional qualifications to get higher than the bottom strand of rope. Nepotism, thankfully, is passing away as a criterion for preferment. But the ambitious supervisor still faces many problems. Not least is his reduced status as a manager. Although nearest the problems and, therefore, in an ideal position to prevent and to resolve grievances, he often finds himself unable to do so. Many supervisors complain of a lack of support and understanding from higher management. Relationships are not improved when decisions, taken according to agreed procedures, are over-ruled by superiors for reasons which are often difficult to understand and are not always explained.

But, if the situation above the supervisor has changed, that below him has also altered radically. Companies can no longer take loyalty and obedience for granted. Rising educational standards and income levels have lifted expectations. People's attitude towards authority has changed fundamentally. The cultural climate demands the flow of communications upwards as well as downwards. Work groups are no longer prepared to be fully committed to the achievement of objectives in which they have had little or no say. The supervisor, even if he had the power, can not afford to treat the workers in his group as 'hands'. The 'hands' have become organized, and some have worked themselves into such a strong bargaining position as to be able to earn as much as, if not more than, the supervisor who has responsibility over them. In days past, the workers' representative, the shop-steward, sorted out problems with the foreman. The foreman had power and authority to act. In the modern situation the shop-steward may still have to talk to the supervisor about problems, because the grievance procedure demands it, but the negotiations that really resolve issues will take place higher up the network, leaving the supervisor to find out later, perhaps from the shop steward, what new agreements have been reached.

All too often one comes across a supervisor who has been appointed to his first-line managerial position solely on the grounds of his record as a shop-floor worker. It is not uncommon for men to leave work on a Friday as fitters or turners and become foremen on Monday morning. So low is commitment to adult training in some companies that the consequence of this action is often to lose a good workman and make a bad manager. When this happens unnecessary tension and conflict can ensue. Frustrations, on both sides, can build up until one day, after what appears to be quite a casual incident, the whole works comes to a stop and the men walk out on strike.

The following comment came from a supervisor, and many others would share his point of view:

'Middle management seem to bend over backwards to keep pace with the unions, giving the opinion that the word of a supervisor doesn't stand for very much. The general feeling seems to be, "I have a job to do; all right, I'll do it and no more. Why should I bother? No one else seems to."'

He outlined four causes of stress in his firm; frustration at being unable to maintain an even flow of work owing to bad planning, lack of communication between departments, lack of promotion opportunities and an absence of any kind of incentive to do well.

'There is no link,' he went on to say, 'for closer working owing to managerial reluctance to meet and talk with persons concerned. Weekly staff meetings take place at senior level where complaints are aired between departments but no improvement takes place. The lot of the production worker has improved greatly, but the position of the production supervisor is getting more difficult.'

Stress can occur anywhere in an organization, but it is most likely to be at its highest in supervision. Another man, recovering from a nervous breakdown, expressed his work problem very succinctly, 'The foreman stands between what management must have and the men don't want.'

Chapter Nine

ALLEN'S AND BROWN'S

Senior management at both companies were approached in the spring of 1972 about the possibilities of doing some research among their production and non-production supervisors. There were three basic aims. The first was to identify the stress symptoms of the two groups in each firm. The second was to explore the possibilities, using statistical methods, of correlations between stress levels and various factors in the working situation. The third aim was to suggest possible ways of reducing or preventing stress at work in the companies concerned.

Several problems emerged right at the beginning. One was how to distinguish between those suffering from stress at work because of domestic rather than working factors. A decision was taken to resolve this problem simply by asking those taking part in the research to indicate if they felt their stress was caused more by domestic rather than work factors and to eliminate their data from the correlation exercises. Just over a quarter of those taking part eventually were shown to come into this category.

Another problem was that of confidentiality. A form of wording was drafted to be printed on each questionnaire. It read, 'The information contained on this form is completely confidential. A report will be produced summarizing the findings from the research but under no circumstances will anyone but the researcher have access to the individual documents nor will it be possible to identify any particular person from the report.' To protect the supervisors still further they were given the option of signing the document, initialling it or leaving the space for identification completely blank. In the event, by far the majority chose to sign or initial their questionnaires and this made personal feed-back to them that much easier.

A questionnaire was designed to collect the necessary information with several linked questions in it to test for accuracy. Approval for the research was given and the work begun.

There was 100 per cent response from Allen's and an 80 per cent response from the larger Brown's. Work was done in the smaller firm first to test the questionnaire and the research methods. Out of all the forms returned only one was rejected as dubious. This high standard may have been due to the quality of the relationship already existing between the researcher and the men and women involved.

Details of the stress levels and the stress patterns in the two companies has already been given in Chapter Six. The job factors considered for a possible correlation with stress were: Age, Length of Service in the existing job, Experience as a Supervisor, Qualifications, Training, Degree of Change, Job Descriptions, Shift Work, Overtime, Demand rise and fall, Back-log of Work, Travel, Responsibility, Numbers Supervised, Rewards and Achievement, Communications with those above Supervision, Communications with the Supervised, Conflict, Lateness, Accidents, Absence, Smoking, Drinking and a variety of Personal Factors such as worry, confidence, enjoyment in the job and sensitivity. Quite a lot of information was collected about training needs, the most time-consuming tasks, lies and dislikes, disciplinary problems, the basic skills lacking in the people being supervised and home factors relating to work.

Enough time has now gone by for the situation in both firms to have changed. A study now would reveal a different picture, but many interesting factors emerged from the original research which deserve a wider circulation. It is not intended to imply that the conclusions reached at Allen's and Brown's have universal significance. Much more research has to be done before anyone gets anywhere near establishing Stress Laws. Perhaps, because of the variables involved, that situation may never be reached. But other organizations may benefit from catching a glimpse of what was happening at two contrasting firms at a particular point in time.

The Age Factor

The age distribution at Allen's and Brown's at the time of the research was as follows:

Age	Allen's % Production	Allen's % Non-production	Brown's % Production	Brown's % Non-production
Under 25	—	—	—	—
Between 25 and 34	6·7	40·00	24·5	41·4
35 and 44	33·3	30·0	37·7	27·6
45 and 54	53·3	30·0	34·0	20·6
Over 54	6·7	—	3·8	10·3

The study showed a decided correlation between stress and age. There was evidence in all the groups of supervisors that as age increased, stress decreased. All those who came into the very severely stressed category were either in their late twenties or mid-thirties.

As a group, Allen's production supervisors were much less stressed than their counterparts at Brown's. At Allen's 60 per cent were aged 45 and over compared with just over 37 per cent at Brown's. The age distribution among the two non-production groups was very similar, with the stress level at Allen's a little higher than that at the other firm. In three out of four groups of those whose stress was caused more by personal or domestic problems rather than work the same trend was observed. It will be seen that neither company had supervisors under 25 years of age, nor were there many in the Over 54 category. One hypothesis to be drawn from this is that companies who have a large number of their first-line managers in the lower age ranges can expect to have to cope with stress problems. Newness in the job, the first years of marriage, mortgages, young families, personal expectations and other factors may well contribute to this situation.

There are a number of ways in which companies might cope with this problem. One is to give training about stress, what it is, how it can be recognized, the medical and preventive treatment that can be given, and to be aware of the likelihood of damage to one's health and career if action isn't taken. Company medical staff, or the supervisors themselves, could be trained to keep a check on stress levels, particularly among those in the early months of new and challenging responsibilities. Young supervisors could be encouraged to talk about their problems with older and more experienced colleagues and practical support given to them to help them through their difficulties.

It is possible that there are other periods in a supervisor's life when help needs to be offered; in middle-age, when problems for men can be as acute as they are for women and in the period leading up to retirement. A chapter in *Occupational Health Practice* (edited by R. S. F. Schilling and published by Butterworth in 1973) entitled 'Mental Health of People at Work' and written by Dr. Alexis Brook of the Tavistock Clinic in London, goes into this problem in greater detail.

The Length of Service Factor

Every new situation is likely to bring with it feelings of vulnerability and apprehension. The transition from school or college to work or the change from one job to another are two areas where stress symptoms are commonly displayed. Of the newly appointed supervisors at Brown's 30 per cent came into the severe or very severe stress categories. Both high and low stress levels were found among those with less than two years in supervision and moderate stress in all four groups among those with between two and five years' service. No evidence emerged to link very severe stress with long service. The link between stress and service would seem to be that the more service you have the less the stress will tend to be. Some evidence for this view was found in two of the four groups.

Irrespective of age, the lesson from this part of the research would appear to be for colleagues and more senior management to give positive support to supervisors especially in the first twelve months of their work.

The Experience Factor

Supervisors with the most experience either at Allen's or Brown's or in previous jobs elsewhere tended to appear in the two lowest stress groups. The moderately stressed group was almost entirely made up of people with between three and ten years' experience. There was little real evidence, though, of a link directly between stress and experience. This might be explained by the fact that experience does not entirely depend on the time factor. A person with ten years' experience as a supervisor might have grown steadily in knowledge and expertise throughout the whole period. Someone else with the same length of experience might have learned little after the first year and ended up with twelve months' experience ten times.

A balance between experienced and inexperienced and young and more mature supervisors would appear to be the goal at which to aim. At Allen's, with 60 per cent in the 45-and-over age groups, the company could count on a wealth of experience in its production departments. A long-term objective there might be to look for suitable replacements to avoid a dramatic loss of skill and a possible increase of stress in five to ten years' time.

The Qualifications Factor

The supervisors were divided into five groups: those without any qualifications whatever; those without a paper qualification but having served an apprenticeship; those possessing a certificate indicating a City and Guilds standard of training; those with Ordinary National or Higher National Certificates and those with diploma or degree qualifications.

At Allen's, three out of four production supervisors without qualifications appeared in the two lowest stress groups. Half those with O.N.C. or H.N.C. qualifications were moderately stressed. No unqualified person came into the severe or very severe categories.

At Brown's, unqualified production supervisors were found in all five stress groups, but 40 per cent of them came into the no or very slight stress category. One person with Group 4 qualifications, i.e., O.N.C. or H.N.C. standard, was moderately stressed.

There were very few production supervisors at Brown's with certificates to indicate a higher than City and Guilds standard of training, but the trend there was similar to that at Allen's. The unqualified were much less stressed than those with certificates or diplomas. The distinction, so far as stress was concerned, between the qualified and the unqualified was even sharper among the non-production supervisors. All the unqualified appeared in the two lowest stress groups. A number of supervisors with higher qualifications showed little or no stress, but they were very much in a minority.

Asked if they would want to be doing their job in another five years' time, several of the more qualified supervisors in the higher stress groups answered in the negative. Perhaps this gives a clue to the link between qualifications and stress, particularly for production personnel. The more qualifications a man has the higher, perhaps, will be his expectations of promotion and advancement.

The major lesson for companies would appear to be to try to ensure that the best use is made of supervisors' skills; that men are not overstretched by being put into jobs way beyond their capabilities, nor under-used by being held back in situations way below their potential. This assumes, of course, that the production situation remains fairly static and that there is an adequate supply of men and women around to fill the vacancies that occur. Both Allen's and Brown's probably feel that they can cope with the situation as it is, but, should major technical or organizational changes be required, both firms, heavily reliant on past experience at the moment, could find themselves under great pressure to up-date their supervisors' formal training. Perhaps both companies need to ask some searching questions. What kind of business are we likely to be in in five years' time? What organizational changes do we anticipate? What kind of supervision will be required? What training programmes are necessary to enable us to achieve our objectives?

The Training Factor

The section in the questionnaire on training brought some interesting results.

Questions were asked about training received prior to appointment as supervisor, since becoming a supervisor and whether the training had been very helpful, helpful, not very helpful or of no help at all. Specific questions were asked about training received in Industrial Relations, Problem Solving, Working with groups and Psychology. Those taking part in the research were asked to indicate areas where they felt further training was required. Answers were assessed and weighted to indicate the level of training needs and the totals compared with each supervisor's stress level.

Three-quarters of those with very little or no training needs had very slight or no stress levels. Of those with high or very high training needs 71 per cent were either moderately, severely or very severely stressed. At Brown's the correlation between increasing training needs and increasing stress was particularly evident.

Among the production and non-production groups at Allen's, 60 per cent and 50 per cent respectively expressed a need for further training in one or more areas. The three leading training needs for the production supervisors were: Industrial Relations, Psychology and Problem Solving. Those for the non-production group were: Problem Solving, Industrial Relations and Management Techniques.

At Brown's 70 per cent of the production supervisors and 76 per cent of the non-production supervisors expressed a need for further training in one or more areas. Psychology, Industrial Relations and Problem Solving were the leading subjects for the first group and Management, Problem Solving and Psychology for the second.

The emergence of Management as a leading training need for both non-production groups was, perhaps, the most significant result, indicating a not unusual practice within industry of appointing people to managerial situations without prior management training. The questionnaires showed that, at Brown's, three-quarters of the non-production supervisors and two-thirds of their production colleagues received no supervisory training prior to taking on their responsibilities.

The high incidence of supervisors expressing training needs at Brown's indicated not only a need to provide pre-appointment training, but to tailor training programmes to meet individual needs.

If inadequate training leads some people into stress situations a setting out of the ten basic steps in training might help those wishing to attack the stress problem from that angle.

Step One – Where are the needs and what are the priorities? What are the critical areas? Where are we likely to get the most return for our training effort?

Step Two – Are the methods we are using the right ones? Does the system need changing? If we give training in area A to person X will it help him to make a better contribution towards the achievement of objectives and towards his own job satisfaction?

Step Three – What is the occupation we are looking at? What does the Job Description say? Is any training specifically laid down? What knowledge, skill and attitude are required on the job?

Step Four – Who are the people to be trained? Is everyone to be trained? Or just a few? Or just one key person who will then go on to train others? What relevant information is there from the last performance appraisal?

Step Five – What are the objectives which we want to be achieved? What do we expect the trainee(s) to be able to do after the training and to what standard? How will achievement be measured? What cost savings can we reasonably anticipate, say, in the twelve-month period following the training? How do these savings compare with the actual cost of the training?

Step Six – What should be the content of the syllabus? (This depends on identifying the training needs and objectives.)

Step Seven – How is the programme to be designed? How can the learning be caused? Who is to do what, when, where and how?

Step Eight – Implement the training programme. Monitor the training. Question the techniques used and improve on them if possible. Get people into action and encourage them to relate back what they are learning. Help those who learn at a slower rate than others.

Step Nine – Review the training. Were the objectives achieved? What was successful and what caused the success? What were the difficulties and what caused them? How do we use what we have learned in order to build on the successes and overcome the difficulties?

Step Ten – Follow-up and evaluate the training on the job. Has the person been able to put learning into practice? Is good progress being made towards the objectives and standards set prior to the training? What else needs to be achieved?

The Degree of Change Factor

It was possible to work out from this section of the questionnaire job situations where there was no change, slight change, moderate change, considerable change and complete change.

The degree of change for the production men at Allen's was slight, but, for their non-production colleagues at the time of the research, almost everything was in a state of flux. It was significant to find people in the midst of considerable change in both the lowest and the highest stress groups. A similar situation was found at Brown's, but, here, there was additional evidence that those whose jobs were not changing at all were, as a group, subject both to high and low stress. Overall, there was some evidence that, as change increased, stress also increased, but it was clear from the distribution of results within each of the five stress groups that the degree of stress resulting from the degree of change was very much a function of the person concerned rather than the amount of change.

If further research should support this hypothesis, then there could be good reason to doubt the often-heard sayings, 'Nobody likes change' and 'A change is as good as a rest'. Change, for some, will produce stress; for others, it might lead to a reduction in stress. No change, for some, will lead to increased stress; others will not appear to be troubled at all.

The lesson to be learned by those implementing change is to recognize those most likely to be stressed by change. The worst stress consequences might well be avoided by taking a little more time in explanation, encouragement and support with such people.

The Job Description Factor

The possibility of a link between stress and job descriptions was investigated. The following questions were asked: Do you have a job description? How does this describe the job you do, i.e., accurately, fairly accurately, not accurately at all? Have you yourself a pretty clear grasp of the job you are supposed to do?

Evidence from Allen's showed that the absence of a job

description tended to be associated with the higher stress groups. At Brown's, half the production supervisors in the lowest stress group, did not have job descriptions but, nevertheless, had a pretty clear idea of the job they were supposed to do.

The Shift Factor

Shift working was a factor to be found in all the stress groups from no stress at all to very severe. It affected production supervisors more so than the others. If anything, the balance was in favour of shift work being associated with the lower rather than the higher stress levels.

The three major problems created by shift work were: dislocation of family life, dislocation of social life and lack of proper sleep. Out of the 22·6 per cent of the production supervisors at Brown's who said that their stress problems were caused more by personal or domestic circumstances than by work, three-quarters were shift workers.

The relationship between stress and shift-work, particularly night-shift-working, may well be an indirect one, except in the case where it interferes with sleep. A person who cannot get used to sleeping during the day will not be able to restore enough mental or physical energy to maintain a high level of efficiency during the period he is working when his body wants to be sleeping. Digestive troubles may well compound the problem. Primary and secondary stress symptoms may well begin to show. If a person can sleep during the day, he may find that his pattern of working so dislocates his domestic and social life that his stress has its source there rather than at work. Each individual then has to choose whether to continue working shifts or look around for another suitable job. It may or may not be possible for a sensitive manager to recognize and respond positively to a situation where he is continually losing good supervisors because of personal and domestic problems caused through shift-working. While it may be possible for him to find permanent night-shift jobs, permanent day-shift working may be completely out of the question except for a very limited number. Ultimately, labour and transport problems may force a firm to abandon night-shift working altogether and look towards other methods of maintaining productivity.

The Overtime Factor

Supervisors were asked, 'How often, on average, do you have to work overtime during the week?' Four or more days per week was considered excessive. There was clear evidence at Brown's that many hours of overtime were being worked by the production supervisors and a clear correlation between increasing overtime and increasing stress was evident. This was also true for the other three groups. When asked why they worked such long hours it was discovered it wasn't simply because the firm expected them to do so; some, for a variety of personal and other reasons, wanted it that way. The mental and physical consequences were all too clear.

For the non-production groups the problem wasn't so much the overtime worked at work but the overtime worked at home. At Brown's, 65·5 per cent, and at Allen's, 70 per cent, said they took work home and, for a third and two-thirds respectively, this was a regular occurrence. Comparative figures for the production groups were much less, but, at Brown's, in addition to the hours worked at work, 40 per cent took work home. Two-fifths said that this was a regular practice. Not surprisingly, their wives had something to say. Of the production supervisors at Brown's 68 per cent said that their wives complained about their spending too much time at work and another 62 per cent said that their wives complained that they were overworking. The incidence of domestic criticism was much, much less at Allen's.

The Department of Employment *Gazette* (published by Her Majesty's Stationery Office) for February 1974 showed that 53·4 per cent of all operatives working in mechanical and marine engineering worked an average 8·9 hours overtime in the week ending 15th December, 1973. The total average hours overtime worked for all manufacturing industries, excluding shipbuilding and ship repairing and maintenance workers, came to the same figure for that particular week. Figures for the amount of hours worked nationally in the engineering industry by supervisors were not stated but the data given did indicate the size of the problem.

Figures produced annually by the International Labour Office in Geneva in their *Year Book of Labour Statistics* show that, in Britain, we not only work longer hours than most other European countries, but succeed in producing less per man per hour. Why this should be is a complex issue involving investment in up-to-date machinery, basic rates of pay, manpower and machine utilization, planning, training and motivation in management as well as trade unions. With all our experience behind us we ought to be able to organize our resources better but we appear incapable of doing so. All too often extra manpower and extra overtime are turned to as means to solve production problems as though organizations were oblivious to the law of diminishing returns and the human and social costs of working long hours, or were afraid of facing up to the basic organizational issues producing the need for so much additional effort. Method Study experts have long been saying that what we need is not men to work harder or longer but men to work better.

When overtime has become endemic in a company so that management and worker alike expect it as part of the normal routine, and, perhaps, feel they could not survive without it, the task of radically reducing it becomes far from easy. But stress, in places where management and men work long hours, could be reduced 'at a stroke' by cutting overtime and helping men and women to make better use of time spent at work and at leisure.

The Back-log Factor

The inability to get work done within the time expected produces back-log and back-log is often the reason for overtime working.

Among the production supervisors at Allen's there was fairly strong evidence that a regular back-log of work was linked with a high level of stress; 75 per cent of the people in this group felt there was a need for better planning in their departments. Presumably, with better planning one could look for a more even flow of work and less stress.

At Brown's, 65 per cent of the production group complained of a regular back-log and as many as 89 per cent felt there was a need for better planning. Among the non-production supervisors at Brown's the proportion of those with a regular back-log was even higher, at 70 per cent, but only 26 per cent of the group felt that planning was a problem. Asked whether they felt that the job was 'getting on top of them', 34 per cent of the production men and 24 per cent of the non-production supervisors answered, 'Yes'. Yet there was really no conclusive evidence of a correlation between back-log and stress. The less stressed groups had the least incidence of back-log, but their position was only slightly better than the highest stress groups. Apart from the production group at Allen's, regular back-log appeared to be a problem more for the moderately stressed. One explanation might be that back-log, like overtime, can become an accepted part of the system and lose some of its power as a stressor. By pinning the blame for back-log on others; the planners, the purchasers, the maintainers of the machines, the recruiters, the trainers and the production controllers, so one is able to live with, and rationalize, one's inability to achieve. This could account for those who had a regular back-log, but no apparent stress. Or one could worry about back-log and become moderately stressed in the process by not being able to clear it away, or one could work like the Devil to avoid a back-log and become highly stressed as a result.

Apart from planning, other factors to emerge which could, conceivably have a marked effect on back-log, were: material shortages, machine breakdowns, inadequate manning and poor machine utilization. A company working hard to reduce these problems could cut back on back-log, reduce overtime and lower stress levels. There is not likely to be an easier way.

The Travel Factor

In all but one group, the non-production supervisors at Brown's, there was strong evidence that the farther away one lived from work, the less the stress. Of the production supervisors at Brown's who lived within a mile of work, 62 per cent were in the severely stressed category. Of those in the two lowest stress groups 38 per cent lived more than ten miles from work and a further 24 per cent between three and ten miles. One explanation could be that, provided your job does not entail a lot of travelling, the journey from work to home gives a person either an opportunity to work off his frustrations on the car or upon other road users, or, by forcing him to concentrate on his driving, helps to take his mind off work problems. As one middle-manager confessed, 'I'm human again by the time I get home.'

There would seem to be some sense in encouraging people under pressure at work not to live 'over the shop'.

Other Job Factors

In addition to change, job descriptions, shift-working, overtime, back-log and travel, several other questions were asked in this section of the questionnaire.

Three questions concerned the matter of overlap with other supervisors and the kind of problems created by this. Outstanding for the production men at Brown's was the recurring problem of communication. This indicated a need for a much better system of communication between the members of this group.

The supervisors were asked to state what were their most time-consuming tasks. Allen's production group listed planning, paperwork, progressing work through the department and problem solving as their four main time consumers. Their non-production colleagues gave problem solving, paperwork, allocating jobs and materials and communicating as their main items. At Brown's the production group listed paperwork (including written reports), progressing work, dealing with machine breakdowns and material shortages as their top four. Their non-production counterparts had paperwork, planning, problem solving and checking work in the department. Paperwork, of one kind or another, came high in all the groups; a task which might be devolved to others in a job enrichment programme. The two production groups showed a high production orientation in their actual work. The group at Allen's were much more involved in planning than those at Brown's.

A team looking into the possibilities of improving work satisfaction would require information of this kind in order to find out what basic duties needed to be retained, what could be passed to others, where the major training needs were likely to appear and what changes were required in the organization to permit the type of supervision desired to come into being.

The supervisors' main likes and dislikes were identified. Allen's production group listed problem solving, achievement, involvement with people, good working relationships and practical work as their top five likes. The non-production group listed achievement, clearing back-log, involvement in projects, new work and freedom in methods of working as their main likes.

At Brown's, the production supervisors gave achievement, working with people, challenge, training others and practical work as the items they most liked doing and their non-production colleagues listed achievement, planning and processing, supervision and problem solving.

Achievement stood out in all the groups as one of, if not *the*, most liked aspect of work. It was interesting that money featured in only one list, in ninth place.

Sensitive managements, faced with lists like these, could encourage their men to develop the things they liked best about work. Perceptive and forward-thinking managers might succeed in developing their subordinates in skills which existing circumstances prevent them from practising: skills which are performed by specialist staff such as personnel managers, industrial relations officers, accountants and training officers, or others at higher levels of line management. Given the motivation to achieve, the possibilities are endless.

The lists of dislikes made interesting reading.

Allen's production supervisors gave industrial relations problems, disciplining, rush orders, poor communication and paperwork as their main ones. Industrial relations problems also came first in Allen's non-production group, followed by, clerical work, disciplining, failure and politics. Brown's production group listed disciplining, paperwork, shift work, constant overtime and differences of opinion as their main dislikes. There were only two dislikes from their non-production colleagues: routine clerical work and poor communication.

The involvement of supervisors in what they dislike doing is more likely to produce stress than involvement in issues they like to tackle. Help given to men to reduce what they dislike doing in order to let them get on with what they like doing must have a beneficial effect. In every position of responsibility people have to face both what they like doing and what they dislike doing. It will always be so. But supervisors do respond positively when support is given in the situations they dislike. Ways can be found to relieve supervisors of a lot of routine paper work, but the chances of avoiding industrial relations or disciplinary problems are negligible. Clear, written, agreed, effective procedures are essential. Maintenance of those procedures, once agreed, is basic if the supervisor is to prevent his position being eroded. Practical training, preferably on a joint basis with worker representatives and more senior management, is a must. If problems are to be avoided supervisors have to be released from some aspects of their production progressing or routine administration in order to see ahead and lay plans for unexpected crises. Only in this way will the stresses, produced by aspects of work which the supervisors dislike but which their responsibilities force them to undertake, be reduced.

Taking the factors of change, job descriptions, shift-working, overtime, back-log and travel together under a general heading of Job Needs it was possible to work out a correlation with stress levels. The supervisors in the lowest stress group tended to have the lowest Job Needs. There was fairly strong evidence among the non-production supervisors at Brown's that as job needs increased so did stress. In every group, supervisors in the very severely stressed category had higher job needs than those with little or no stress.

A comparison of Job Needs and Training Needs showed that people with high Training Needs almost invariably had high Job Needs. Some supervisors with low Training Needs also had high Job Needs. The hypothesis suggested by the study is not, if you train people well enough you will eradicate job needs and minimize stress levels, but rather, if you do not train people well enough job needs will develop and stress will increase.

The Responsibility Factor

This section of the study dealt with numbers being supervised, increases and decreases in responsibility, willingness or otherwise to accept more responsibility, boundaries of responsibility, overlapping of responsibilities, lines of authority, staffing and actual responsibilities such as recruitment, training, dismissal, assessment, discipline, and dealing with grievances.

A number of interesting factors emerged. One was that none of the supervisors in the very severely stressed category had more than what could be called 'average responsibility'. Although three of the groups statistically showed some evidence of a correlation between increasing responsibility and increasing stress, the evidence wasn't very strong. In each of the five stress categories, from no stress at all to very severe, supervisors with relatively low levels of responsibility appeared side by side with others with relatively high levels. The responsibility results were similar to those in the section dealing with the degree of change; suggesting that whether responsibility causes stress or not depends not so much on the actual weight of responsibility but on the manner of its coming and the personality which receives it. Although more than a third of the production group at Brown's did admit to feelings that, sometimes, their job was 'getting on top of them', more than 90 per cent of the total number of men and women in the research, when asked, 'Would you be prepared to accept more responsibility?' answered, 'Yes'. Douglas McGregor's Theory Y proposition that the average human being learns, under proper conditions, not only to accept but to seek responsibility would appear to be borne out by this study.

The supervisors were asked, 'How many people do you supervise?' They were divided into five groups.

Group one   –   1 to 3 people
Group two   –   4 to 6 people
Group three –   7 to 14 people
Group four –   15 to 24 people
Group five –   25 people and over

In both production groups there appeared to be some evidence that as the size of the numbers supervised decreased, so stress increased. The correlation between decreasing size and increasing stress was very marked among the non-production supervisors at Brown's. Supervisors with three or less people to supervise were all in the moderate to very severely stressed categories. Half those with between four and six people came into the top three stress groups. Supervisors in the third group, i.e., those with between seven and fourteen people to look after, were spread fairly evenly across the stress categories, but 62 per cent of those with fifteen to twenty-four and 58 per cent of those in Group five appeared in the unstressed or slightly stressed categories. Having to cope with large numbers was a problem for some, but these were very much in a minority.

The data pointed to the conclusion that stress was most likely to be a problem for supervisors of very small groups rather than for those responsible for large numbers.

When particular situations were considered the reasonableness of this hypothesis became obvious. In data-processing, small groups of people operate their computers on a shift-work basis. Perhaps there are just three people shut up together in a relatively confined space, one of whom is the team leader. Relationships in such situations can become intense. Interpersonal difficulties, particularly in times of sustained pressure when dead-lines have to be kept, can have serious consequences. If one member of a team of three fails to turn up for work, unless a replacement can be found, the work-load on the two remaining increases by 50 per cent. On the other hand, if a supervisor is responsible for forty men working on a line of machines, he cannot possibly get to know them all very well. It is unlikely that relationships, especially if there is a continual turn-over of personnel with new people having to be trained every other week, will ever develop beyond the superficial. If, out of the forty, one man fails to clock-in, the increase in work-load is negligible compared with that of the computer team. The thirty-nine can, usually, manage quite well: with a little re-organization.

The selection of supervisors is a difficult business at any time, but companies need to be particularly careful when appointing men and women to be responsible for small groups. Some experience and skill in working with others as a team and some understanding of behavioural problems would appear to be essential requirements for those accepting such a responsibility. A withdrawn, autocratic, non-participative type of supervisor could be the worst possible choice.

All the supervisors had responsibility for discipline; one of the aspects of working life least liked by all four groups. The production men at Allen's put lateness, time-keeping, poor quality work and absence as their leading problems. Allen's non-production group also had lateness in first place, followed by 'discussion groups', 'sickness' and lack of interest in the job. The production supervisors at Brown's produced exactly the same list as their contemporaries at Allen's and the remaining group of non-production supervisors at Brown's said that their leading causes of disciplining were: lateness, idle chatter, absence and lack of attention.

The similarity across all the groups was remarkable; and

disturbing. Reading through the lists of problems one recalled an article in the November–December, 1972 issue of the *Harvard Business Review* by Richard E. Walton, Edsel Bryant Ford Professor of Business Administration and Director of the Division of Research at the Harvard Business School. The article was entitled, 'How to counter alienation in the plant' and his main thesis was that, faced with fundamental changes in the expectations of employees towards themselves, authority, work, organizations, advancement and the American competitive way of life, and the decreased productivity and increased social cost caused by a perpetuation of traditional organizational forms, nothing less than a total, systematic restructuring of the way work was done would counter the fact of employee alienation. His list of symptoms included: job dislike, personal resentment, rebellion against the union, reduced concern for quality, withdrawal, absenteeism, increased labour turn-over, inattention, pilfering, sabotage, deliberate waste, assaults, threats, bombings and disruption. Walton questioned the willingness of managers to undertake the major innovations necessary for redesigning work organizations to deal effectively with the root causes of alienation.

The evidence produced by the supervisors at Allen's and Brown's did indicate a growing state of alienation among employees. If Richard Walton is right, and recent organizational development at the Saab-Scania plant at Södertälje and the Volvo complex at Kalmar, Sweden, would appear to support his view-point, then supervisors have little hope of reducing their problems over discipline by superficial means that do not attack root causes. Without a willingness for fundamental change their problems, and their stresses, are likely to continue.

The Rewards and Achievement Factor

Questions in this section were asked about pay, promotion, appraisal, career prospects, changing jobs, standards of performance, recognition of achievement, criticisms and complaints.

The worst possible situation was conceived as being one where a supervisor was receiving inadequate pay both with respect to responsibilities and personal needs, felt that promotion prospects were poor and deteriorating, was without regular appraisal, had no one with whom to discuss his career development, was worried about falling standards of performance in the department, had a boss who rarely recognized achievement and was unhelpfully critical about insignificant things.

The results showed clearly in all four groups that as rewards and achievement declined stress increased. No one ran up a maximum adverse score but 90 per cent of the production supervisors and 75 per cent of the non-production group at Allen's appeared to have problems along with 64 per cent and 55 per cent respectively of their counterparts at Brown's.

Asked if they felt they were adequately and fairly paid for the responsibilities they bore at work, about 50 per cent in each group answered, 'No'. When asked, 'Is your pay adequate for your basic personal needs?' dissatisfaction at Allen's appeared to be much greater than at Brown's; 26·6 per cent of the production group and 30 per cent of the non-production supervisors at Allen's registered dissatisfaction compared with 9·4 per cent and 13·8 per cent at the other firm. It was interesting to discover the slightly higher dissatisfaction about pay among both non-production groups, though the problem appeared to be due to higher personal needs rather than disagreement about levels of responsibility. The pay problem at Allen's was reflected in the response to questions about changing jobs. The incidence of supervisors seriously thinking of moving on was 7 per cent higher at Allen's compared to Brown's.

Mention has already been made in Chapter Eight about the lack of promotion opportunities for supervisors. Of the two groups at Allen's only 13 per cent of the production men and 10 per cent of their colleagues in non-production felt that their chances of promotion at the company were good. About 40 per cent altogether felt their chances were not good and the remainder simply did not know. At Brown's a slightly higher proportion were optimistic; 18 per cent and 28 per cent respectively. But 32 per cent of the production group and 44 per cent of the non-production group were pessimistic and 50 per cent and 28 per cent respectively did not know.

Allen's appeared to have a problem in both areas. Promotion opportunities seemed greater at Brown's, perhaps because of their size, but favoured the non-production group much more than the production men. The relatively high level of people in three of the groups who just did not know about their future career prospects suggested the need for improvement in career appraisal.

The way the supervisors felt about promotion was revealed by their answers to the question, 'Have your promotion prospects improved during the year?' – 93 per cent of the production group at Allen's and 80 per cent of their non-production colleagues said they had not, or that they did not know. The corresponding figures at Brown's were 74 per cent and 76 per cent.

The proportion of production supervisors prepared to take promotion to a more responsible job were 73 per cent at Allen's and 72 per cent at the other company. Among the non-production groups, 70 per cent and 76 per cent respectively were willing to move upwards.

The data showed a situation where a majority wanted promotion but were dubious of getting it. Such a situation must cause frustration.

A company might tackle the problem in a number of ways. It could decide, as a matter of policy, that promotions be from within. It could make certain that promotion ladders, with opportunity to receive suitable training for advancement, did exist. It could raise the status of supervision by delegating responsibilities to supervisors from higher levels of management and relieving them of duties capable of being carried out at lower levels. Companies could provide facilities for discussions about career development. They could avoid raising expectations to an unrealistic level. A stress-conscious Personnel Manager might even encourage an ambitious and capable supervisor to move to another firm where opportunities for advancement could be brighter. It is possible that a future society, based on self-supervision and project teams, could scrap the whole idea of pecking-orders and encourage employees to relate to one another more in terms of what they can contribute towards the achievement of group objectives. White coats, names on office doors, numbered places in the car-park and separate canteens for each section of the work-force would then be irrelevant.

Uncertainty at Allen's about supervisors' prospects probably arose partly out of inadequacies in the firm's appraisal system. At the time of the research only 13 per cent of the production group had had regular appraisals and none had discussed their career prospects with anyone. By comparison, 55 per cent of their counterparts at Brown's had appraisals and 18 per cent had discussed their career prospects during the previous year. The non-production group at Allen's fared much better with 60 per cent having had appraisals, but this fell short of the record shown by Brown's non-production supervisors, 93 per cent of whom were appraised. There were more discussions, too, about career prospects among the non-production groups. The respective figures were 30 per cent and 41 per cent. But there was little evidence of continuous appraisal. For the most part, appraisal exercises appeared to be of a once-per-year kind.

With achievement figuring so highly in the lists of the things most liked about work in all four of the groups at the two companies, it would appear that both Allen's and Brown's could benefit greatly by supplying regular feed-back about performance. A continuing appraisal system could identify successes and their causes and build on them. It could also pinpoint difficulties and their causes and create opportunities to overcome them.

About 40 per cent of the non-production supervisors said that their bosses complimented them regularly for achievement. Only 20 per cent of the production groups received this kind of praise. In addition, the latter groups received twice the criticism about 'insignificant things' than their opposite numbers in non-production. Overall, the picture was one of low and, often, negative, feed-back; a situation which would cost little or nothing to remedy. The consequences of recognition for real achievement could be very creative.

But the problems were not restricted to lack of recognition for achievement. The supervisors also commented about the basic skills lacking in the men given to them to do the work. At Allen's the production group said they lacked experience, theoretical approach, basic mathematics, ability to make decisions and right attitudes. The non-production list was: experience, technical skill, commercial training, planning skills, the ability to work on their own and right attitudes.

The supervisors at Brown's gave similar lists, but in a different order. The production men gave right attitude to the job, machine shop experience, engineering background, training, ability to analyse technical problems and basic technical skill as the deficiencies they recognized in their people. The non-production list was: right attitude to the job, on-the-job knowledge, experience, theoretical knowledge, effective use of time, ability to think and compatibility.

The lack of experience ranked high in all the groups. Training deficiencies were also very much to the fore. But the most interesting comparison concerned right attitudes. It seemed to be much more of a problem at Brown's. According to the supervisors, having a right attitude to the job included having enthusiasm, confidence, vigour, concentration, perseverance, a sense of responsibility, initiative, drive, diligence, interest, improvisation, 'wanting to know' and the will to work.

A comment from one supervisor was very much to the point, 'The present intake of school leavers shows a marked reluctance of teenagers to take orders or accept any form of discipline. They see no need for teamwork or for any need to work a five-day week. Getting over to the majority any sense of responsibility is very difficult indeed, and will, I believe, get worse.'

This man was not one of the supervisors in the original research but his word would probably be echoed by many in charge of younger people. No doubt the way people are expected to work, the boring jobs many of them do and the poor quality of working relationships they have to endure do affect attitudes. James Lawson's experience in Chapter Seven is a good example of this. But the task of establishing right attitudes is as much society's problem as industry's. It has to do with homes and schools and colleges and universities as well as machine shops and training centres. Careful selection might weed out the worst offenders, but, in a situation where labour is short, even this becomes a difficulty.

Perhaps the beginnings of an answer to the attitude problem does lie with industry; in making absolutely sure that a creative link exists between the world of work and the world of education where basic problems can be aired in a constructive way with headmasters and careers teachers. The churches and the media have also a part to play. The supervisor, too, by word and example, has to take his share of responsibility, if only because he is often the one nearest the problem.

Before leaving this point, it has to be said that the problem of wrong attitudes at work has to do with adults as well as with school leavers. Attitudes which have been developed over long periods of time take long periods of time to change. Nor is it simply a problem to do with individuals. The influence of groups is immense; and this applies to managers as well as to trade unionists. Perhaps the biggest help that companies can give to supervisors is to recognize that people have emotional problems at work as well as technical and organizational ones. If a man, in a leadership position among a group of men, can be given training to recognize when a person has an emotional problem, and if he can be helped to understand what can happen both within groups and between groups, he will be in a better position to respond helpfully when things begin to go wrong for no apparent technical reason. If he is allowed time to tackle the human as well as the technical problems and to plan his work in such a way that unnecessary human or group or inter-group problems are avoided, he may, with skill, patience and persistence, discover he is able to achieve much more than the men who approach their work in a highly production-oriented and authoritarian manner. There is no doubt that such people achieve results over the short term, but they only do so at great cost to productivity and human welfare in the longer term.

Over all the groups there was no case of a person with a high sense of reward and achievement being under anything more than slight stress. There were those who had low levels of reward and achievement in the lower stress groups, but the incidence of such people in the moderate to very severe categories of stress was twice as great. The situation to aim at, therefore, on the basis of the research, would appear to be: reward supervisors adequately on the basis of the responsibilities they bear, give due recognition to personal needs, recognize and reward real achievement, give opportunities for advancement either by real growth on the job or promotion to positions of greater responsibility, appraise continuously, provide positive and helpful feedback, provide the supervisor with adequate resources in order to achieve his objectives, give him help in understanding human and group problems and time to work successfully through them and recognize that a flourishing industry is not likely to emerge out of an unflourishing society. These actions would help to reduce stress caused by problems in this area of work life.

The Communications Factor

There was very strong evidence indeed from three out of the four groups that stress increased as communications problems increased. In this section of the questionnaire supervisors were asked, first of all, about communications with those immediately above them. Questions were put about ability to communicate exactly what needed to be done, whether important messages tended to be left out or not, the speed of follow-up, the appreciation of the supervisor's problems, personal interest, whether or not the reason for doing jobs was invariably given, the degree of checking up once a task had been allocated, availability when needed, the use of first names, the degree of listening, and various other personal factors likely to affect communication such as impulsiveness, readiness to believe rumours, reluctance to accept new ideas and the problem of a superior being withdrawn and difficult to get to know.

Only among the non-production supervisors at Allen's was there evidence to the contrary of a strong correlation between increasing stress and worsening communications. Here, improved communications with higher levels of management led, not to less stress, but to more. This group was, it will be remembered, the most highly stressed of all the groups, and undergoing, at the time of the research, considerable reorganization within the company. With some of the group facing the prospect of possible redundancy, one explanation of their response could be that, when the situation is threatening, good communications can increase the build-up of stress. Having a good communications system with managers who have excellent relationships with their supervisors will not necessarily make for less stress. The stressor in this situation will not be the hang-ups between people but what is actually being communicated. Good news will bring relief. Bad news will cause stress. Where the working situation, therefore, is potentially threatening, the only way to improve the mental health of employees would appear to be for the company to improve its trading position and make certain that there was far more good news to report than bad. In a potentially thriving situation the problem of bad news will be reduced. Good communications will aid the general sense of well-being. Poor communication will become the stressor.

There was overwhelming evidence from both production groups and the non-production supervisors at Brown's that good communications with higher levels of management was a feature of low rather than high stress. There was some evidence that a few supervisors in the two lowest stress groups had managers who were poor communicators, and there was a very small number of supervisors in the severe or very severe stress categories who had superiors who were good communicators but their presence was not great enough to invalidate the basic hypothesis. But it did indicate that, as well as environmental factors, personal factors were also of significance when tackling communication problems.

Out of the two non-production groups, 20 per cent in one case and 17 per cent in the other said that their immediate superiors were withdrawn and difficult to get to know. When faced with a particularly difficult problem, 20 per cent and 14 per cent respectively acknowledged that they tended to keep it to themselves and behave in an introvert manner. There was more than one situation where two introverts were together, supervisor and manager. Not surprisingly, communications between them were difficult. A company, recognizing the importance of personal factors in communication, could encourage introverts to share problems. A sensitive third-party might be able to remove half the difficulty simply by getting two people together to appreciate their similar natures.

If a supervisor believes his boss is confused, uncertain, indecisive, forgetful, slow to respond, interfering, short-sighted, impulsive, rumour-prone, withdrawn, preoccupied, disinterested, unrealistic, insensitive, resistant to change, hostile and a poor listener, the chances will be that the boss is under very severe stress himself and in urgent need of medical help. Nobody in the research assessed their superiors quite as badly as that, but 40 per cent of the supervisors at Brown's with severe or very severe communication problems were, themselves, under severe or very severe stress. In this situation, the supervisor may be able to recognize the tell-tale stress signs in his boss, but, because of his own difficulties, may not feel able to do much about it. He may believe, and console himself with the thought, that it is not his responsibility to discuss personal matters with his superior. But, if his own stress problems are not too great, and if he has the kind of relationship with his boss where they can talk openly together, the supervisor may be the one person in the works who can help his manager to recognize, and take steps to deal with, a stress situation. Admittedly, it is much more difficult for a person in a subordinate position to advise someone above him what to do, but the subordinate, like the secretary who can tell immediately the boss opens the office door whether he is under stress or not, may well be the first one to see, as well as to feel, the boss's stress. There are all kinds of tactful ways of finding out why a job needs to be done or checking that information received has been correctly understood. A manager may or may not have the sense to say to a supervisor, 'Now, just that I can be absolutely sure that you've understood what I want you to do, will you feed back to me what I want you to do?' If he does practise that technique he will always be able to avoid problems arising from misunderstanding or poor listening, but, if he does not ask, politely and non-threateningly, for feed-back, there is no reason why the supervisor should not take the initiative. The supervisor might say, just as his boss is about to pick up the telephone and deal with another problem, 'I can see you are busy, but, just to make sure that I've got all the details, can I quickly run through what I think you want me to do?' The supervisor has only himself to blame if he starts a job only half understanding what it is he has to do. His lack of courage in failing to admit his failure, fully, to grasp instructions at a briefing session will only lead him into greater difficulties later on when a botched job reveals his ignorance.

Clarifying objectives and checking comprehension through feed-back, asked for or volunteered, is a skill all communicators would do well to learn. Equally important for future success is the manager's and the supervisor's willingness to spend a little time at the completion of a task reviewing what went well and why, so that the success can be carried over into the next project, and looking at any difficulties and their causes, so that corrective action can be planned before the next task is allocated. Such a review could look at the human as well as the practical issues. It need not take long. The creative possibilities of regularly appraising a situation in this way are immense. It could lead to continual improvement in performance. It could provide not only feed-back but stimulate sound ideas for overcoming problems. It could identify difficulties at a very early stage. By recognizing success it could lead to a build-up of confidence for the supervisor and his team and for the manager. The question for the manager is not, 'Can I really afford time to conduct such reviews?' but, 'Can I really afford not to review successes and difficulties in this way with my supervisors?'

At both Allen's and Brown's the demand for more openness from managers was very significant. When asked, 'Do you feel there is a need for a more open attitude about company issues by managers?' 79·8 per cent of the production group and 80 per cent of the non-production group at Allen's said, 'Yes'. The answers in the affirmative were even higher at Brown's; 85 per cent and 82·7 per cent respectively.

The second section of the questionnaire dealt with the quality of communications between the supervisor and those whom he supervised. The questions asked of the supervisor about his manager were rephrased slightly and now put to him. The results showed, quite clearly, that there was an association between good communication and low levels of stress. The correlation between worsening communication and increasing stress was quite marked in the production supervisors at Allen's and the non-production group at Brown's. The non-production group at Allen's conformed, this time, to the general pattern. Overall, the supervisors rated their ability to communicate with their workers rather lower than their ability to communicate with their managers. The production men at Brown's appeared to be the poorest listeners. They had the highest impulsiveness rate and were the only group to call for more openness from the men on the shop-floor than from their managers. Among their non-production colleagues only half had regular meetings with their staff. The same proportion confessed to not receiving a constant flow of creative suggestions from the people they supervised and they had four times the incidence of tending to keep problems to themselves.

The data showed that it did not always follow that a supervisor who had little difficulty communicating with his boss had the same level of success with his workers. Similarly, those who had problems with their superior did not always fare as badly with those they supervised. But, among those with severe or very severe stress, the tendency to have communication problems all round, that is, with both boss and worker, was much more noticeable.

At Brown's the supervisors in the production areas had difficulty not only in communicating effectively with their managers and their workers but with one another. 'Communications' was almost unanimously identified as the major recurring problem across the group. Meetings between all the production supervisors at Brown's were difficult to arrange because of their three-shift system. At Allen's, a company operating a day and a night shift only, lateral communication was not so much of a problem.

Communication problems appeared to fall into three main groups. Firstly, problems arising because of inadequacies in the communication itself, i.e., the word spoken, the instruction, the memo. Secondly, problems arising out of some environmental difficulty, for example, an awkward shift-system or the absence of a regular group meeting to discuss matters of common concern. And, thirdly, problems arising out of personal and inter-personal or group and inter-group difficulties. This section could range from: lack of courage to admit to failure to understand fully what is being communicated; inability or unwillingness to listen, through lack of openness and lack of trust, to deliberate withholding of information in order to repay some injustice or maintain a position of power over someone else. The solution to the first two types of communication problem may well be difficult, but not too complicated. Resolving the other type may well be a complicated and drawn-out business. On the whole, industry appears to do well on the technical and straightforward issues. It is rather less adept at handling situations with a high emotional content.

Following the research, a group of supervisors was called together for an exercise in listening and understanding. This was intended to be a first step in improving communications. Each member was asked to come prepared to discuss a particular communications problem in the group. The leader determined beforehand that the group should do the bulk of the talking and that he would only interrupt in order to draw out key issues and help the group to achieve its objective.

After the initial introductions the leader displayed a chart on which was written, 'The aim of this session is to help you improve your ability to be heard and understood.' The aim, expressed in terms of their need, helped to gain their commitment and, as a *rapport* developed between the leader and the group, he outlined the programme for the session and indicated some approximate times for each stage. When the leader felt that he had gained the commitment of the group to the aim he asked the supervisor on his immediate left to present his communication problem. This having been done, he turned to another member of the group and asked him if he would like to feed back to the others the problem as he had heard it. Questions were asked to draw out key details. Other members of the group then added their comments. The process was repeated around the group; problems were presented, played back and clarified. In almost every case the problem played back differed from the problem presented. 'Third parties' helped to shed new light on each situation. Throughout this part of the exercise the leader observed the group at work and watched for the connected conversations that would indicate the degree of listening. He encouraged the quieter members of the group to contribute to the discussion and tried to hold back the more eager ones. The clarified problems were charted and the main types identified. Problems arising out of personal or inter-personal difficulties were clearly dominant and the leader asked the group to consider how, within the working situation, the supervisors might overcome this type of problem. Each person was encouraged to express his point of view and the leader checked for comprehension among the others. The group looked at the problem of getting feed-back in a non-threatening way from subordinates and giving feed-back to management, and how to cope with a variety of 'emotional' situations. The final exercise of the session involved the group splitting up into pairs and one person finding out from his partner what practical lesson had been learned during the session. Everyone then stated what they had gleaned from their partners and this was checked and cross-checked. Not only were members of the group able to check their ability to be heard and understood but the final exercise provided useful feed-back for the leader on the effectiveness of the whole session. Checking for listening and comprehension continued right up to the end.

In any communications situation human factors will continually appear to thwart perfect listening and understanding. The shop-floor is no exception. A listener will make his own selection from and put his own interpretation on what he sees and hears. But, by putting himself in the listener's position, by watching how his words are being received and by obtaining feed-back in a non-threatening way, a communicator may be able to avoid many problems. It is unlikely that communication skills will come easily or without a lot of practice or without a lot of care being given to developing relationships of trust, openness and respect within which people are able to receive without misrepresentation and feel free to question without fear of being humiliated.

The Conflict Factor

A supervisor cannot avoid conflict. He stands at the point of implementation. Upon him rests responsibility for getting things done; for the realization of plans and decisions in which he may have had little or no involvement. He may have to allocate work loads to people who have little motivation to work and one dominant thought in their minds; the wage packet at the end of the week. The supervisor's task can generate inner conflict, strain working relationships, cause friction at home as he gives vent to his frustrations, build up resentment, create grievances which may or may not be dealt with quickly or effectively, raise ethical issues and stimulate strong objections to company policy and administration.

The questions in this section of the questionnaire were devised to establish the level of potential stress in the situations faced by the supervisors. There was very strong evidence of a correlation between increasing conflict and increasing stress among the production men at Allen's and the non-production group at Brown's. The evidence was less conclusive among the production supervisors at Brown's where men with fairly high degrees of conflict were to be found in all five stress categories. But, even here, 43 per cent of those with 'severe' conflict had severe stress. In every group, low levels of conflict were associated with low levels of stress.

With few exceptions those with severe or very severe stress had a high incidence of worry. Of the non-production group at Brown's 31 per cent had conscience problems. This, in fact, was the lowest percentage among the four groups. The group with the highest figure was Allen's production men with 41·4 per cent. Worry about work ranged from 20·7 per cent among the non-production supervisors at Brown's to 70 per cent of the non-production section at Allen's. Of this latter group 80 per cent also worried when work was not done on time. Only their colleagues in production had a higher score, at 86·5 per cent. Levels at Brown's were lower at 56·6 per cent for production and 51·7 per cent for non-production. Allen's non-production supervisors headed the groups on worrying when disciplining (60 per cent). They were the most frustrated (50 per cent). They showed the highest level of dissatisfaction about the solution to work problems (60 per cent). They were the most dissatisfied about company policy (70 per cent); levels elsewhere were around the 40 per cent mark. Along with their production colleagues they showed the strongest resistance to change (40 per cent). They had the biggest incidence of lying awake at night after being criticized (40 per cent). They had the strongest resentment at being by-passed (40 per cent) and the greatest feeling that shop-stewards were more a hindrance than a help (50 per cent). Yet, in spite of all this, an examination of levels of conflict against levels of stress showed that as conflict reduced over the group as a whole, stress increased. Compared with their production colleagues, who had fewer worries about disciplining or work, were much less sensitive to criticism, less resentful, the least dissatisfied of all the groups about the way work problems were handled, the least perturbed about company policy and the least bothered about work 'getting on top' of them, the non-production supervisors at Allen's had twice the level of stress. The results from this group showed, as did all the others, that low stress can be a feature of both people with low and high levels of conflict. In this case those with high conflict levels were concentrated in the no-stress to moderate-stress categories. These supervisors represented 62 per cent of the group. Two-thirds of the remainder appeared in the top end of the moderately stressed category and in the very severely stressed category: the other third, representing 12·5 per cent of the total group, being in the lowest stress category.

The evidence pointed to a number of conclusions about the relationship between conflict and stress. The fact that a person shows little or no sign of stress is no proof that he has little to worry about at work. He may have a high sense of work satisfaction and general well-being and, therefore, little stress, or he may have a lot of problems, but, because of his way of handling conflict, in a positive and open way, he may manage to keep stress to a minimum. A group that faces up to problems and works through them may find that they are able to handle conflict without it becoming too much of a stressor. The next best thing to having a situation where everyone is satisfied may be to have a creative approach to conflict. This may explain why it is possible to have high conflict and low stress.

High levels of conflict and high levels of stress might come about through the unrelenting pressure of continuing dissatisfaction. A group may try hard to resolve problems in an open, but unsuccessful, way. Alternatively, stress may well be produced by problem avoidance. A group may have problems but owing to an inability, perhaps, to organize themselves properly to handle their difficulties, or an unwillingness to face up to them, they may find themselves in a stress situation. In both these situations continuing work dissatisfaction and conflict will tend to create more and more stress.

The situation remains of the person with low job dissatisfaction and high stress. His problem may be one of avoidance, but, more likely, the stress may point to the fact that the absence of conflict in an organization may well be an indication of low job dissatisfaction but not necessarily a sign of high job satisfaction.

The clue, then, to the link between conflict and stress may well lie not so much in the amount of conflict but in the manner in which it is approached in the company. Organizations may find that the best way to reduce stress is to encourage employees to bring their problems, their worries and fears, out into the open where they can be discussed and dealt with in an understanding and effective way. The setting up of speedy grievance procedures and the provision of training in problem-solving would appear, from the research, to be as important for a company's managerial employees as for its shop-floor workers. At Allen's and Brown's more than 50 per cent of the supervisors wanted a greater say in the resolving of industrial relations problems.

The Smoking Factor

A remarkably high 60 per cent of supervisors at Allen's were non-smokers. There was no evidence that those who smoked more than twenty-five cigarettes a day did so because they were under severe or very severe stress. At Brown's the heavy smokers tended to be among the lower stress groups, but 44 per cent of the supervisors there did say that their smoking had increased during the year, and, with two exceptions, all showed signs of stress.

The Drink Factor

Only at Brown's was there evidence that drinking increased as stress increased. No questions were asked directly about alcoholism, but recent estimates suggest that between 3 and 5 per cent of any given work-force are thought to be suffering from the illness with a third of that number in the later stages of it. The cost to British industry is thought to be in the region of £500 million through lost performance, efficiency and productivity. Companies, such as Allen's and Brown's, ought to be alert to the drink factor and know where the nearest centre for the treatment of alcoholism is located. Timely help and advice might save problems at a later stage.

The Personal Factor

Worry was, undoubtedly, a significant factor in the build-up of stress. The main source of worry appeared to be when work was not done on time. This was a particular problem at Allen's where there was 30 per cent more worry about this than at Brown's.

The research also showed that the supervisors who liked things exactly right almost invariably had stress symptoms.

There was some evidence from both production groups that, as stress increased, so supervisors lost confidence. An overwhelming number, when asked if they enjoyed their jobs, answered in the affirmative. For a small percentage enjoyment tailed off when stress was high, but it was also clear that severe or very severe stress did not preclude enjoyment for everybody. The degree of sensitivity to criticism was almost six times as high among the non-production group at Allen's compared with their production colleagues. This may well have contributed to their high average stress level.

The Home Factor

Although the main emphasis in the research was on the working environment, some examination of the domestic factor was undertaken. Home factors were the main stressors for a third of the production men and a fifth of the non-production supervisors at Allen's and for 22·6 per cent of the production group and 31 per cent of the non-production section at Brown's. Altogether, only 9 per cent had more than moderate stress while 48 per cent showed no or very slight stress signs. Though significant, the results underline the importance of the working environment when it comes to identifying the causes of supervisors' stress problems. Organizations, such as the Church, which concentrate much of their activity in the domestic sector of society might take note of this fact.

When asked if they received support and understanding at home about problems at work, the production men at Allen's gave the highest affirmative response at 86·5 per cent. The lowest figure, 77·4 per cent, was returned by Brown's production group; 68 per cent of Brown's wives complained that their husbands spent too much time at work. This was more than twice the proportion of the wives of Brown's non-production supervisors and five times greater than the figure for Allen's production group. Wives' complaints about overworking showed a similar pattern, except that Brown's production supervisors appeared to suffer ten times the criticism borne by their opposite numbers at the other company. Complaints at home about worry about work were highest, at 80 per cent, among the wives of the non-production group at Allen's. Elsewhere, the figures were around the 33·3 per cent mark.

The supervisors were asked, 'Do you find it easy to leave all thoughts of work behind when you go home?' At Allen's 46·7 per cent of the production group said, 'Yes.' Of the production and non-production supervisors at Brown's 45·3 per cent and 38 per cent respectively also said, 'Yes.' Not a single one of the non-production group at Allen's felt able to answer in the affirmative. When asked, 'Do you find it easy to leave domestic issues behind when you come to work?' the figures were much higher – 80 per cent of Allen's non-production group said, 'Yes', as did 79·3 per cent of their opposite numbers at Brown's. The figures for the production groups at Allen's and Brown's were 60 and 68 per cent respectively. This highlights, again, the impact of the working environment on a person's life. The figures suggest that the best returns on investment in a programme for the improvement in a working man's mental and physical health are most likely when the problem is tackled from the industrial and commercial end.

Summary

Some interesting correlations between stress and various factors in the working environment at Allen's and Brown's emerged from the research.

The most highly stressed were in their late twenties or mid-thirties. A course of training about the problem of stress, personal counselling and practical help with problem solving might aid such a group.

A third of the newly appointed supervisors showed severe stress symptoms. This suggests a need for special support during the first twelve months in a new appointment.

Those with qualifications tended to have more stress than those without. Getting a better fit between personal abilities and job requirements might help here. A realistic discussion about future prospects could be a further aid.

Inadequate training led to stress situations. Training tailored to individual personal and job needs could be one way to overcome this problem.

Change was stressful for some, but not for all. Identifying those likely to be most adversely affected by change and taking appropriate action might reduce the effect of this stressor.

Having a clear idea of the job helped.

Shifts dislocated family and social life and patterns of eating and sleeping. People with problems at home might find shift-work leads to increasing stress. A change of job may be the only way out of this difficulty.

There was a clear link between overtime and stress – the more the overtime, the more the stress. A cut-back in overtime and the taking of work home could have a very beneficial effect.

Back-log of work created stress. One way through this

problem could be to have better planning and a more efficient use of resources.

The nearer a person lived to work, the greater tended to be the stress. This problem might be solved by encouraging supervisors not 'to live over the shop'.

Achievement stood out as the factor most liked about work. Recognizing and rewarding real achievement should be a key feature of management.

Industrial relations problems and disciplining emerged as principal job dislikes. Proper training, the setting up of effective and agreed procedures and the maintenance of those procedures until better ones are drawn up could help to take a lot of the stress out of this situation. Support from higher management would appear to be essential.

Small groups had high stress levels. This would appear to call for careful selection of leaders of small groups, and for some training in group dynamics.

Increased responsibility caused stress problems for some, but not for all. A careful allocation of responsibility would help here.

Alienation between supervisor and supervised was evident. To overcome this stressor might call for a major organization change after the pattern of the Saab-Scania plant and the Volvo complex in Sweden.

There was plenty of evidence that stress increased as rewards and achievement declined. Pay, promotion and appraisals are key factors to consider in this area.

A right attitude to the job was a key missing factor among men at work in Allen's and Brown's. This problem cannot be solved by industry alone. A much better liaison has to be established between managers, unions, teachers, careers officers, local authorities, community groups and parents.

Poor communications led to increased stress in most cases. Basic exercises in listening, getting feed-back, and learning how to review performance with a view to improving both what is done and how people relate to one another in achieving objectives could be of major help in reducing stress problems arising out of poor communication.

It was felt that managers needed to be more open with their subordinates and workers more open with their supervisors.

There was some evidence that increased conflict led to increased stress. It was also clear that avoidance of conflict led to increased stress. By bringing problems out into the open where they can be dealt with in an understanding and effective way stress levels might well be significantly reduced.

Increased smoking could be a sign of stress.

Increased consumption of alcohol could be a sign of stress.

Worry played a significant part in the build up of stress.

For the majority, what happened at work was more of a stressor and less easily shrugged off than what happened at home. This would appear to point to a need for increased effort at work to understand stress and its causes and to set in motion changes within the working environment to reduce stress levels.

Home factors played an important part in those with stress at work. The influence of these factors should not be ignored.

Chapter Ten

WHAT CAN BE DONE ABOUT STRESS AT WORK?

If there is stress at work, it will show. The person under stress will feel the aches in the jaw and neck muscles, the prolonged indigestion, the recurring headaches, the anxiety, the tension and the other primary symptoms that characterize life on the wrong side of that ever fluctuating threshold between ability and inability to cope. Others will sense the stress in a wide range of secondary symptoms that could include increased smoking and drinking, changes of mood, withdrawal, indecision, out-of-place aggression, absence, proneness to accidents, delayed recovery or persistent behaviour change. As the stress increases, efficiency and productivity will suffer. Those nearest the man or woman under stress will sense it first. The consequences will quickly rub off on to others.

There are no quick and easy solutions to the kind of stress problems that arise out of the working environment. Organizations, and the groups and people who operate in them, are extremely complex creatures. The attempt to do something about the problem of stress at work by bringing certain contributory factors out into the open may, in fact, increase stress for some. This may be the emotional price some organizations have to pay before a patient working-through of difficulties or, maybe, a severance of relationships, creates a less stressful situation. There is no guarantee, either, that, after the expenditure of vast sums of money on a new plant lay-out or a management development scheme, stress will not persist at work. Man, as well as being part of a complex working system is, at the same time, part of a complex personal relationships system and part of a complex economic and governmental system. He may also be, for good measure, part of an ethical system that sees man as much more than an extension to a machine or, after forty years, a disposable cog in a profit-making process. But the view that every man, whatever his class, colour or creed, has a value and dignity and a right, not just to work, but to health and life, may be the one liberating factor that persuades those who have responsibility for the way organizations are run to embark on the risky business of reducing stress at work.

Much could be done without the expenditure of vast sums of money.

More publicity could be given to the prominence of mental ill-health in sickness absence. *Off Sick*, the report produced by the Office of Health Economics in 1971, which showed that nervousness, debility and headache and psychoneuroses and psychoses were the second and third fastest growing causes, respectively, of sickness absence in Britain between 1954–5 and 1967–8, was based on statistics already held by the Department of Health and Social Security in London. If the changing pattern of days lost through strikes can be monitored, there is no reason why days lost through mental ill-health should not be given similar treatment.

Training programmes on what stress is, how it is caused, how it can be recognized and what the first steps might be in reducing stress levels, should not be too difficult to set up. According to the Press Notice issued by the Department of Employment when the Health and Safety at Work Act received the Royal Assent at the end of July, 1974, the Act 'provides the most comprehensive ever system of law covering the health and safety of people at work and the public at large who may be affected by the activities of people at work'. The Health and Safety Commission to be appointed under the Act 'will have a research, educational and advisory role and will be responsible for the continuing job of preparing proposals for revising, updating and extending the statutory provisions on health and safety at work and for issuing approved codes of practice'. Furthermore, the Act will provide for the continuation of an Employment Medical Advisory Service, which, in addition to a number of specialists at Headquarters, one of whom will have special responsibility for mental health problems, will have fifty-two full-time and forty-two part-time doctors in nine regional centres. Under the Act the E.M.A.S. advises on the 'safeguarding and improvement of the health of people in employment'. It also has authority to investigate problems with which it is concerned. When the service was first introduced early in 1973, the then Secretary of State for Employment, Mr. Maurice

Macmillan, wrote, 'For the first time there will be within the Department of Employment a nation-wide service of specialist doctors who will be able to give advice about the medical aspects of employment problems to workers, management, trade union officials and other doctors. It will deal not only with industrial diseases in the narrow sense but also with the strain and tensions arising from modern technological society.'

Here, at least, was recognition of the importance of the mental aspect of health at work.

Yet another body that could help in the process of education, training and prevention is The Society of Occupational Medicine. On 1st October, 1973, this organization had 962 members representing doctors in a wide range of industries and other places of employment.

According to the Department of Employment News No. 12, a total of 450 works medical officers had been appointed by the beginning of 1974 to 'carry out statutory periodic medical examinations of workers engaged in hazardous trades'. There were sixty-five occupational health nurses included in the service and based mainly in Skills Centres and Industrial Rehabilitation Units run by the Department.

The factory doctor should be brought into the training programme at work. He may be a member of the Society of Occupational Medicine, and have had some training in this field though the chances are that he will be a very busy General Practitioner with limited O.M. expertise and little time to understand the complex circumstances that cause stress at work. In their evidence to the Roben's Committee on Safety and Health at Work the British Medical Association stated that out of 2,000 factories employing more than 500 people only 1,300 had the services of a part-time or full-time doctor. Out of 195,000 factories with a hundred or less employees, about 1,800 had visits from a part-time or full-time doctor. Commenting on the 1,500 Appointed Factory Doctors the B.M.A. said that few of them spent more than a very small part of their time on A.F.D. duties and few would claim any particular expertise in occupational medicine.

The programme of training about stress at work ought to include some guidance on personal counselling. Managers, trade union officials and shop stewards should be encouraged to develop a skill in this field; their work often requires it. All too often a person with a problem is sent to a Personnel Department and to 'specialists' who are remote from the situation where the problem arises. The man, taken out of the situation, finds himself in a strange environment among people he does not know and who do not know him. Not knowing how far he can trust those to whom he has been sent, he may only feel able to reveal part of the problem, or no part of the problem at all. Well-meaning fellow employees in the remote office are not able to help him and the problem remains unsolved. Only when it is accepted that training, industrial relations, problem solving, development, welfare and other similar aspects of the Personnel Function are a part of the Job Description of every manager – and training provided in these areas – will industry be able to solve its problems in the best way: as and when and where the problems arise. One of the good points of the Code of Industrial Relations Practice, drawn up by the Conservative Government in Britain in the early 1970s, was the recognition that the supervisor was a key person in problem-solving simply because he was the representative of management nearest the problem.

The work at Allen's and Brown's suggested that there was a link between inadequate training and increasing stress. A five- to ten-year programme aimed at improving management skills might, indeed, be costly, but, if the result is better counselling, a better fit between personal aptitudes and job requirements, training for those who need it, help for those adversely affected by change, reduced overtime and back-log through better planning and a better use of resources, a better feed-back about real achievement, effective and well-maintained procedures, a fair payments and promotion system and an open, trusting and creative relationship between manager and manager and manager and managed, the benefits could far outweigh the training costs.

The fundamental problem of making such a change might not be finding the money for such a programme but persuading managers to learn entirely new behavioural skills. The problem was aptly summed up by K. Robertson in his article on 'Managing People and Jobs' (*Personnel Management*, Sept. 1969). Comparing participative management with more authoritarian forms, Robertson defined the former as 'the discipline whereby an organization learns how to tap something of the latent potential of its members. It involves entirely new skills of behaviour; it requires from managers a whole new understanding of the processes that happen both within and between groups of people. It is, in fact, the gradual, stressful, risk-taking process of experience by which management matures from its out-moded role of directing, controlling and governing to its new role of enabling, encouraging, assisting and reinforcing achievement by others.'

The attempt to change from one type of management style to another may be one of the stress increasing factors mentioned earlier. Some managers, including supervisors, may feel very threatened indeed by such a change. They may resent giving up duties and responsibilities they have come to regard as their own. They may feel too old to change to new ways of working. They may fear redundancy. They may band together in unions to protect their positions.

If a company does look for more creative and less stressful ways of working the risks involved in developing a more participative system may be just as great for union representatives as for managers. Some unions have been brought up on a tradition of vigorous and active opposition to employers; seeing themselves as a permanent opposition, accepting what is in their interests and resisting what is not, rather than a potential government or partner in government. The abandonment of the old system, with its frequent confrontations resulting in a win or a loss for one side or the other, and its replacement by a more participative system, where each side wins, could result in a shop steward coming into conflict with the traditionalists in his union and losing his office as a result of their thinking he had 'gone soft'.

An organization which wants to do something about stress at work and wants to tackle root causes must take such matters into consideration. The problem is not just one of financial feasibility, but human feasibility.

Some organizations will find that training people to adapt to the system will not overcome the stress problem and that the only way forward is to adapt the system to fit in with the people. Volvo's immensely bold and highly costly decision to scrap the assembly-line method of building vehicles in preference for a more personally satisfying group scheme may well have set a pattern for other companies trying to cope with problems of alienation, absenteeism and labour turn-over.

Peter Drucker, in his book *Technology, Management and Society* sums up this particular problem. 'All institutions,' he says, 'will have to hold themselves accountable for the quality of life and will have to make the fulfilment of basic social values, beliefs, and purposes a major objective of their continuing normal activities. We will become far less concerned with "management development" as a means of adapting the individual to the demands of the organisation and far more with "organisation development" to adapt the organisation to the needs, aspirations and potential of the individual.'

In addition to training about stress at work, the solution to the problem may require a fundamental change both in the behaviour of managements and unions and in the way institutions are organized.

Assessing the Problem

Many difficulties surround the problem of dealing with stress at work. Confused thinking has equated stress with pressure and this has led to the view that stress is necessary, in some way, if objectives are to be reached on time. The mental aspects of health at work have, until recently, been given little prominence. Denied proper guidance in handling stress problems, management and unions have adopted a *laissez-faire* attitude. Doctors have prescribed treatment but without a real understanding of the environmental pressures at work. Statutory bodies, under the Health and Safety at Work Act, have hardly begun to get to grips with the problem. Not all companies have had the courage, or the financial resources, to embark on costly reorganization programmes. Yet the problem persists and appears to be growing. Some writers, among them Alvin Toffler, think that between now and the beginning of the next millennium millions of psychologically normal people will experience an abrupt collision with the future. In his book, *Future Shock*, he argues that many will be unable to keep up with the supercharged pace of change and will be brought to the edge of breakdown by incessant demands to adapt to novelty. He describes the symptoms of future shock as ranging from confusion, anxiety and hostility towards helpful authority, to physical illness, seemingly senseless violence and self-destructive apathy. Among other signs he includes erratic swings in interest and life style, followed by panicky feelings that events are slipping out of control and social intellectual and emotional withdrawal.

It was not a finding of the research at Allen's and Brown's that people under stress at work tended to take positive steps to deal with basic problems. Out of the seven supervisors identified as being under very severe stress and in need of urgent medical help, four had not been to a doctor at any time during the previous twelve months. Every member of this group ran considerable risks of a mental or physical breakdown.

Every company knows just how dislocating the unexpected loss of a key person can be, not to mention the costs involved in finding a suitable replacement. For what it would cost to recruit, induct and develop a person to take over a job suddenly made vacant because of the breakdown of a man or a woman under stress, companies could keep a watch on levels of stress within the organization. A screening process might prevent a health breakdown for someone.

A small firm might feel a need to approach an outside body, such as the Employment Medical Advisory Service, for help. Larger organizations might ask their medical adviser or a member of his or her staff to undertake the task of screening. Given the willingness of the people involved to co-operate, the job itself need not be difficult. It will be necessary to say something about stress and the purpose of the exercise. Confidentiality may be a problem for some and assurances will have to be given about this. Some precise instructions will need to be given about what and when and how to record the information required.

An example of a Stress Analysis Form is given at Figure 8 in Chapter Five. This, when completed, will provide information about:

    a person's name and age

    title of job

    number of years in present job

    main responsibilities

What can be done about Stress at Work?

most time-consuming tasks

major work problems

an indication of whether a person is having treatment from a doctor or not

an indication of the main source of stress

a list of stress symptoms from which a score and grading can be obtained

date completed and location.

When completing the form it is important that the stress symptoms (if they exist) should reflect how a person is feeling, or felt, in a given situation, say, at work, and at a particular time, for example, during a morning or afternoon or night-shift.

Information about how to score and grade the form is given at Figure 7 on page 53. If the scoring and grading is not being done by the person filling up the form, time should be set aside for a confidential feed-back of information to those requiring it. A person with no stress symptoms may feel he or she ought to have some! A person with a low grading may want to discuss a particular problem. Those with moderate or higher gradings should certainly be seen. Those with very severe stress should be encouraged to see a doctor.

A completed set of forms will provide an individual stress pattern for each person. If a particular occupational group has been involved, a stress pattern for the whole group can be worked out by adding up the various symptoms and ranking them in order of incidence. The more varied the group the less significant will be the stress pattern for the whole group.

The information may show that a particular occupational group, for example, the shop stewards or the computer operators or the female supervisors, was showing a particularly high stress level at the time the data was collected. This could indicate a problem common to all the members of the group. Plans should be laid to undertake a further investigation in such circumstances. Alternatively, the information might reveal that only a small proportion of the occupational group were showing signs of moderate to very severe stress. In any one group of twenty-five people it is normal to expect at least one person to be showing very severe stress symptoms. In this case, a decision has to be taken whether to involve the whole group or only a few individual members of it in the follow-up.

If stress levels are low, with no one with a count of more than eight or nine, it may be felt that the situation does not warrant further action at this stage. The position may be reviewed after a further survey at a later date. On medical grounds it may be felt that the level of stress is not too serious. On company grounds it may be felt that some of the problems listed on the left-hand side of the stress analysis form do warrant attention.

This raises the question of who decides what follow-up action to take. If the screening is approached on a purely medical plane important industrial or organizational issues may well get overlooked. An assessment panel comprising a doctor, a senior executive and a small number of management and employee representatives may be part of the answer to this problem. A joint group of this nature may, on looking at all the information, decide to press for action on a number of work problems, irrespective of whether a serious stress problem exists or not. If this is the feeling of the group after one or more surveys, and feedback to individuals involved, the assessment of the stress problem can be said to have entered a critical phase.

Follow-up

Follow-up can be through individual action, action involving others, or both. Where the sources of stress have a high personal content – see Chapter Two for some examples – a sympathetic and understanding counsellor may be able to encourage a person under stress to take effective action to reduce his stress level himself. He may, for example, be able to suggest courses of further training, ways of delegating responsibility, people who would give help if asked, how to gain commitment from others, how to go about solving problems, how to set realistic objectives, how to get feed-back from others, what to stop doing in order to concentrate on the really important things and so on. It will be necessary for a counsellor to keep a confidential record of problems raised, plans laid and action taken for reference in subsequent conversations. If a counsellor can establish a relationship of trust and confidence with the person under stress and can get that person to talk frankly about the problems producing the stress then there is hope for improvement. A few

What can be done about Stress at Work?

positive steps could produce a lowering in the level of stress. But where stress arises as a result of workplace or organizational problems, or problems to do with the industry, or technology, or economics, or commercial pressures, individuals, on their own, with or without a good counsellor, cannot bring about quick and effective change.

Follow-up action that, of necessity, involves others will always be more difficult than that which can be initiated by one person and controlled by that person and seen through to a successful conclusion.

At the factory level the problem solving approach which involves joint action by the important interest groups would appear to be one way of initiating change with an ultimate objective of reducing stress and increasing job satisfaction and all-round health and well-being. But, given the will among managers and trade unions jointly to work towards a situation which will achieve such an objective, authority to make radical changes is often limited for both. Trade Unionists have to work within rules and managers within systems where authority and power is often vested in Boards far removed from local plant level. The decision radically to alter a manufacturing process or to revolutionize management styles is normally not one that is taken at local level. Managers and trade union officials often have to work with one hand tied behind their backs; the organization and the culture prevailing within the organization limits their freedom, but this is no valid reason for not using the freedom that does exist to create the organizational conditions within which human growth of men and women at work becomes possible. The person or group campaigning for reduction of stress at work has to take note of the political and organizational forces that are to be found in any large enterprise. Their research has to be good; their arguments well-founded. They have to be prepared to use every line of communication and every relevant power group to make their voice heard. They have to keep at it, patiently and creatively. Some important international companies have taken action and spent large sums of money to root out soul-less working systems. As concern grows and understanding of what stress at work can do to a man, and to the organization for whom he labours, others must follow.

Help From Others

The need for change lies at the heart of the stress problem. The individual is not totally without freedom to influence his environment. It was the Psalmist's belief that man had been made 'little less than a god', crowned with 'glory and honour' and made master over all God's creatures. It is part of the tragedy of modern humanity that man has only aspired to be just a little bit better than the Joneses. He has pursued work in order to make money in order to keep one step ahead in material goods. He has lost the vision of creative work. He has forgotten the art of sharing wealth and skills with the poor. He campaigns for the right to work, but not for the right to health and life. There is a sense in which stress at work, and in society, is largely man's own creation. He has been duped into believing that the good life lies via the way of acquiring consumer goods. Others have played on his innate belief that work is, in some way, an essential part of the dignity of man, by forcing him to labour in meaningless ways. Soul-less work has gradually destroyed millions of those made little less than a god. It has rendered them incapable of enjoying either wealth or what that wealth can buy. Organizations have stifled initiative and creativity. It is significant, not that workers sometimes rebel, but that they do not rebel more often.

Part of the blame for this sub-human condition must rest with the guardians of faith and ethics who have courted the wealthy and neglected the poor, preached the necessity of work and remained silent about the enjoyment of life, counselled obedience to authority when it would have been better to have stood, like the Tolpuddle Martyrs, and fought. Changes in management or trade union styles or in organizations will not come about without a revolution in man's appreciation of himself and his world. If the guardians of faith and ethics will not speak out and if men and women cannot be found to share in the decision-making processes in a way that upholds the value and dignity of man the radical changes that are required to improve the health and well-being of people at work will never occur. The moral aspect of the stress at work problem is not a peripheral issue; it is central, seminal, fundamental; one of the major liberating influences that can enable industrial man to challenge and change the *status quo*.

What can be done about Stress at Work?

The school teacher and the adult educationist have an important role to play. A survey conducted by the Department of Education and Science of Careers Education in Secondary Schools in England and Wales in 1971 and 1972 reported that many schools were not effectively in touch with the working world. 'Careers education', the report said, 'is concerned explicitly with preparation for adult life and with the acquisition of knowledge and development of skills which have relevance for the future. Implicit in the continuous process are: self knowledge; the exploration of the material world and the people who live in it; the training of the intellect; the development of the creative and aesthetic senses; the challenge of moral principle and the response to it; the awareness and understanding of spiritual values.' (p. 61f.) The survey went on to ask for a policy of careers education for all pupils from the age of thirteen onwards; a curriculum in schools that keeps doors open; a pastoral system of which careers education forms an integral part; careers work co-ordinated by a nominated teacher with the necessary training, experience and status; active involvement of other members of school staffs in careers work and effective communication between all concerned with the curriculum and with pastoral care; time made available both for teachers and pupils for careers work; effective working relationships with the careers office, with higher and further education and with the world of employment; adequate collection and storage of information about all pupils; effective discussion between the pupil and all concerned with guidance – parents, teachers and careers officers and adequate accommodation and resources in the schools for this kind of work. Education has to be brought into a closer relationship with the world of work, which, of all the sectors of society, does most to shape the lives and attitudes of people. Teachers have to be encouraged to supplement their career paths which, all too often, begin in school, progress to university or college and end up in school again, with some real experience of what life can be like at work. As well as equipping pupils with knowledge and basic skills – principally in the spheres of English and Mathematics – schools have to help their pupils to understand themselves and the society in which they are living, to improve their ability to communicate, to gain appreciation of the behavioural problems that can arise when human beings gather together in groups, to have some idea of how to solve problems, to develop leadership skills, to learn how to establish and maintain relationships in an adult world, to learn how to survive when that adult world appears neither to want to hear what they have to say nor to care.

Young people in their twenties tend to be among the most highly stressed of all age groups. It is not surprising when the price they have had to pay in pursuit of knowledge has been the failure to prepare properly for living in a rough and often insensitive society.

Adults, after a few years of exposure to working life, become conscious of huge gaps in their education. People at work ought to be encouraged to fill in those gaps and to see education as a process extending over the whole of life. Adult education is needed not just to develop people at work, but to enable them to use their leisure creatively and to play a full part in developing a flourishing society; an essential requisite for a flourishing industry.

Teachers in Polytechnics and Business Schools have also something to offer; principally in the fields of communication and sensitivity training. It is of little use training students in the latest techniques of financial planning or manpower development or industrial relations if, at the end of the course, students lack the ability to get their message over to others and have difficulty forming the kind of relationships within which creative work can occur. A person who is technically competent but unable to relate effectively to others is likely to have a stressful career. One of the biggest contributions managers and trade union officials can make to relieving stress at work is to be good at their jobs. As Doctors Blake and Mouton have outlined in their book, *The Managerial Grid*, this means possessing both a high concern for producing goods and services and a high concern for people.

Governments can give help. They cannot legislate for the removal of stress at work any more than they can legislate for good industrial relations or creative participation between workers and management. Governments have a responsibility, along with bodies such as the C.B.I. and the T.U.C., to set up some national guide-lines to make certain that the pace of voluntary action is both increased and under-pinned. Governments can insist on change and encourage it along the direction

What can be done about Stress at Work?

it must take. The Health and Safety at Work Act and the development of the Employment Medical Advisory Service are good examples of what can be done, but a close co-operation is needed between Governments, managements and unions to ensure that the right kind of improvements are made to the systems evolved so that those systems can respond positively to ever changing circumstances. In the case of stress at work more attention may need to be given and more resources released in order to cope effectively with mental health.

Doctors have an obvious contribution to make in the diagnosis and treatment of mental ill-health, but there are signs, even within the medical profession itself, that a patient-oriented approach to the problem of stress at work is far from adequate. A doctor may feel that his main responsibility is to the person who comes to him for help, but he also has an educational and advisory role to perform. If prevention is better than cure doctors must be encouraged to take time to understand the environmental conditions that produce the mental and physical diseases which, in time, necessitate treatment. It must be in their own interests to try to reduce the flow of patients through preventive medicine and joint consultation with employers and trade unions aimed at improving working conditions. If health at work is to be the fundamental aim, rather than the treatment of ill-health, managers and workers have their part to play in this process as well as the doctor. They need his help to identify where the danger areas are, so that changes can be made. They need some of his insights to be able to recognize tell-tale symptoms, give first-aid in an emergency and know when professional treatment is necessary. All too often situations occur at work where, for lack of elementary knowledge, people are pushed far beyond their coping capacity into areas of severe or very severe stress. The temporary or permanent breakdown that sometimes results, and causes such dislocation in the work and the family environment, might well have been avoided had there been someone around in the factory to spot the problem at an earlier stage.

It is in the interests of shareholders, whether public or private, to make certain that their money is invested in systems that are geared to efficiency and productivity. Stress at work can only impair efficiency and reduce productivity in the long run.

Companies may, by increasing the pressure on their employees, produce impressive results in the short term, but, in time, workers will become organized to resist that pressure with the inevitable consequences of demotivation, apathy, alienation, excessive wage demands, absenteeism, poor time-keeping and increased labour turn-over. No share-holder can be happy with this kind of situation.

Industrial planners and engineers can help by looking not only at the technical attributes of the machines or the machine shops they produce, but what happens to human beings required to work with or in them. In time, no doubt, it will be possible to get machines to do the most mundane jobs and thereby release operators for more creative tasks. Community planners, looking for jobs, may think twice about attracting firms that can only offer employment on machines designed specifically to do one simple task and arranged in such a way that an operator has little need to use his or her mind or little chance of improving innate skills. If local authorities can have second thoughts about the human and social costs of housing families in high-rise flats, they may recognize a need also to examine those working situations which produce so much ill-health and alienation and social apathy.

Not least among the groups that can give help to those working under heavy pressure at work is the family. J. M. and R. E. Pahl in their book *Managers and their Wives* make the point that the drive for greater efficiency at work is occurring at a time when the quality of personal relationships and marriage appear to be on the decline. If this is true then an increase in stress at work can be expected as men and women are denied love and understanding and support from their families. The first signs of stress at work may show themselves in the more relaxed and less threatening atmosphere of home. It is most important that wives and husbands of wives at work should be able to recognize stress symptoms. It is even more important that there should be some understanding of the working situation that may be contributing to the stress problem. A wife who understands something of the problems her husband has to cope with at work through contact with colleagues and their wives, visits to work either for work appreciation courses or special Open Days, or from what her husband tells her, may be able to give invaluable help at the time it is most needed. Her role in enabling him to recognize root causes or getting him to a doctor for effective treatment may be crucial. Children, too, should appreciate some of the problems their parents have to face at work. Unwittingly they can so easily help to increase worry and tension in the family.

Some supervisors at Allen's and Brown's said that they never talked about work problems at home. Some claimed to be able to leave work behind altogether at the end of the day. While one can understand the reluctance of men to burden their wives, who may, themselves, have more than enough to cope with, with extra worry, it is to be doubted whether most men, after a gruelling eight- or nine-hour day filled with problems, can dissociate themselves completely from what has happened, or what may happen in the near future, and be perfectly relaxed and refreshed by the time they arrive home. In a secure, loving relationship, entered into for better and for worse, for richer and for poorer, in sickness and in health, it ought to be possible to talk openly about problems and give support, understanding, help and sympathy one to another.

Conclusion

I was always taught that something which had an Introduction had to have a Conclusion. As an end-piece I want to do two things: to say, briefly, why stress at work concerns me personally, and to pose some questions which, I hope, will open up further discussion.

Most people who read these pages will have been under stress at one time or another. They may have produced good, imaginative and creative work during that period. They may have learned things about themselves and discovered, in others and in society, qualities of life which, in less trying times, may have remained hidden. I take the view that a certain amount of stress is inevitable for anyone taking on responsibilities in the family, at work, or in the community. It cannot be avoided, any more than death – a very stressful experience for most people – can be avoided. But to say that stress is unavoidable or inevitable is not the same as saying that it is necessary. To hear some people talk one gains the impression that, in order to produce work on time, you need a system that promotes throbbing headaches, sleeplessness, depression, anxiety, tension, fear and dread. I don't believe it. In fact, against the creative work done by people under stress I would set what must be a much greater volume of achievement which has been a sheer joy to produce. There are many men and women at work who have high job satisfaction and show not a sign of stress. There are many others, if given a chance by the system to make use of the latent ability that is in them, could have life and have it much more abundantly than they have at present.

I believe stress to be potentially damaging to mental and physical health and to the best-laid schemes of the most financially astute boards of directors. I recognize, particularly in a country so heavily dependent on manufacturing as is Britain, that production has to be maintained and goods sold at competitive prices, but I do not believe that we have tapped anything like the full production potential that exists in British industry. The fault lies in no one particular direction. The lack of investment in modern plant and machinery may be one problem, but there are still far too many authoritarian and inflexible systems that stifle initiative and demotivate effort. Unions, as well as managements, are to blame. I recognize that some systems will have to disappear before real growth can occur and that this will cost a lot of money and necessitate a vast amount of retraining, but I do not accept that it will not be worth it in the long run, nor do I believe that we have to wait for ten years before the economic viability of the ambitious projects some companies have embarked on is proved to the world. Many of the barriers to increased productivity that currently exist could be removed quite simply and cheaply, given a willingness for people at work to relate to one another as human beings.

We cannot wait until all uncertainty and all risk is removed before employers and employees set about changing their behaviour towards one another at work because of the human and social costs of continuing as we are. I happen to believe it would be worth while economically to change and I certainly believe that the social benefits of less stress at work would be enormous. But what disturbs me most is not just what is happening to the economy but what is happening to people. I go a long way with Marxists in their concern to change systems. I would like to see a radical change in the distribution of wealth throughout the world. I firmly believe in the New Testament principle, from each according to his means, to each according to his need. But I do not believe such a change will come about until man faces up to the crisis in himself.

One cannot think about the needs of another if one is totally absorbed in thinking about oneself. Industrial man can change, but he values his authority over others, the continued improvement of his wages and conditions of work and an ever-increasing economic growth more than health, life, justice and a stable social order. He will work all the hours of overtime he can to under-pin an ever-increasing standard of living though he knows that others are poorly paid and unemployed, that more than half the world's population lives permanently on the borderline between starvation and under-nourishment, and that the hidden bonus to his extra effort is a worsening stress problem. It does not make sense, especially in a world where material resources are rapidly in decline and where society is falling apart at the seams through lack of people prepared to accept positions of leadership and responsibility in the institutions that help to maintain its vitality and social cohesion.

Any system is only as good as the people who operate it. The stress at work problem is symptomatic of out-of-date systems and a gross impoverishment in man's understanding of himself and the purpose of life.

I believe that life is meant to be lived and enjoyed; all people, the world over, have a right to health and work and life. How we change from our present unhealthy and unbalanced and highly vulnerable system depends on finding enough courageous men and women to challenge present trends and prepared to involve themselves, sacrificially if need be, with others, to work for a new social and industrial order.

QUESTIONS FOR DISCUSSION

Chapter One
Which of the people described in this chapter do you feel most sympathy for?
How would you set about resolving their problems?

Chapter Two
What are the main stress-producing areas, or potential areas, in your life?

Chapter Three
'A certain amount of pressure appears to be necessary if human beings are to develop and mature and make a creative contribution to society.'
Under what circumstances at work are you at your most creative? At your least creative?

Chapter Four
What stress symptoms are you currently showing at work?

Chapter Five
What is your stress level?
Can you think of any circumstances that have contributed to this condition? (Do the exercise at the end of the chapter.)

Chapter Six
Of the four groups of supervisors studied, the non-production groups in the two firms were much more depressed and had a higher level of stress than their production colleagues.
Can you think of any reason why this should be so?

Chapter Seven
Work affects society and society affects work. What has been the impact of social and industrial change on your part of the world?
How does your working environment influence you at home and in your activities in the community?

Chapter Eight
What trends in relationships between employers and employees (a) do you welcome and (b) do you deplore?
What do you think needs to be done where you work to promote the things that are good for the people who work there and to overcome the things that are bad?

Chapter Nine
Put yourself in the place of the General Manager at Brown's and at Allen's.
What list of priorities would you draw up to improve life at work for each of the four groups of supervisors?
What objectives would you aim at? How would you set about achieving them?

Chapter Ten

What major difficulties have to be overcome before embarking on a programme to reduce stress at work?

Does it really matter what you believe about man and society? What views are currently held at the place where you work?

Does this help or hinder industrial relationships, job satisfaction, achievement, attitudes to work, etc.?

How well do the schools, colleges and polytechnics in your area fit young people and adults for life in a working world?

What might your company or organization do to help develop a more fruitful relationship between education and work?

What further action do you think the Government should take in the mental health field?

Suppose your company doctor said, 'Yes, I know that prevention is better than cure, but I haven't time to get involved in that kind of work.' Would this mean that you could do nothing about stress at work?

How do you think this problem might eventually be solved?

What information should be given to shareholders to enable them to see that a company was being run in a healthy way?

When installing new machinery or designing a work area what could be done ensure that the effect on employees will not be detrimental to their mental as well as their physical health?

What responsibilities have companies to the wives or husbands of employees?

If it helps a wife to understand some of the problems her husband faces at work is there anything a company can do to promote this?

READING LIST

Books

Blake, R. R. and Mouton, J. S. (1964) *The Managerial Grid*, Gulf Publishing Co.
Briggs, Asa. (1968) *Victorian Cities*, Pelican.
Brown, J. A. C. (1954) *The Social Psychology of Industry*, Pelican.
Burns, T. (ed.) (1969) *Industrial Man*, Penguin.
Burns, T. and Stalker, G. M. (1961) *The Management of Innovation*, Tavistock Publications Ltd.
Clarke, R. O., Fatchett D. J. and Roberts, B. C. (1972) *Workers' Participation in Management in Britain*, Heinemann.
Department of Education and Science (1973) *Careers Education in Secondary Schools*, H.M.S.O.
Drucker, P. F. (1970) *Technology, Management and Society*, Heinemann.
Fraser, R. (1947) *Incidence of Neurosis among Factory Workers*, H.M.S.O.
Friedmann, G. (English translation 1961) *The Anatomy of Work*, Faber.
Health and Safety at Work Act, 1974. H.M.S.O.
Herzberg, F. (1966) *Work and the Nature of Man*, World Publishing Co.
Jaques, E. (1951) *The Changing Culture of a Factory*, Tavistock Publications Ltd.
Jaques, E. (1956) *The Measurement of Responsibility*, Tavistock Publications Ltd.
Kearns, J. L. (1973) *Stress in Industry* Priory Press.
King-Taylor, L. (1972) *Not for Bread Alone*, Business Books.
Likert, R. (1961) *New Patterns of Management*, McGraw-Hill.
Maslow, A. H. (1945) *Motivation and Personality*, Harper.
McGregor, D. (1960) *The Human Side of Enterprise*, McGraw-Hill.
Office of Health Economics (1971) *Off Sick*.
Pahl, J. M. and R. E. (1971) *Managers and Their Wives*, Penguin.
Peter, L. J. (1973) *The Peter Prescription*, Bantam Books.
Robens Committee (1972) *Safety and Health at Work* 2 vols. H.M.S.O.
Schilling, R. S. F. (ed.) (1973) *Occupational Health Practice*, Butterworth.

Scott, S. (1971) *Behavioural Theories*, Coverdale Educational Publishers Ltd.
Selye, H. (1957) *The Stress of Life*, Longmans Green.
Toffler, A. (1970) *Future Shock*, Bodley Head.

Articles

Bacot, E. (1972) 'Nature red in ink and tape', *Business Administration* Jan.
Erskine, J. F. and Brook A. (1971) 'Report on a two-year experiment in co-operation between an Occupational Physician and a Consultant Psychiatrist', *J. Soc. Occup. Med.* **21**, 53.
Ferguson, D. (1973), 'A Study of Neurosis and Occupation', *Brit. J. of Ind. Med.* **30**, 2.
Paul, W. J., Robertson, K. B. and Herzberg, F. (1969) 'Job Enrichment Pays Off', *Harvard Business Review,* March–April.
Pettigrew, A. (1972) 'Managing under Stress', *Management Today*, April.
Robertson, K. B. (1969) 'Managing People and Jobs', *Personnel Management*, Sept.
Tyrer, F. H. (1974) 'Have we an interest in Mental Health?' *J. Soc. Occup. Med.* **24**, 1.
Walton, R. E. (1972) 'How to counter alienation in the plant', *Harvard Business Review*, November–December.
Whiting, B. J. (1972) 'Job Satisfaction: reflections on a European Reconnaissance'. Testimony before U.S. Senate Employment, Manpower and Poverty sub-committee, 26th July.

Appendix A

Job factor   *Level of stress*

	Allen's Production	Allen's Non-production	Brown's Production	Brown's Non-production
1. As age increases	D*	D*	D	D*
2. As experience increases	NAC	NAC	NAC	NAC
3. As number of years in present job increases	D*	NAC	NAC	D
4. As qualification increases	I*	NAC	I	NAC
5. As training needs increase	NAC	NAC	I*	I*
6. As degree of change increases	D	I	I*	I
7. As job needs increase	I	NAC	NAC	I*
8. As job demand increases	I	D*	D*	I*
9. As shift-work increases	D	NAC	NAC	D
10. As overtime increases	I*	I*	I*	I*
11. As job description becomes less accurate or is non-existent	I	I	D*	D
12. Regular backlog	I*	D	NAC	NAC
13. As distance between home and work increases	D	D*	D*	I*
14. As responsibility increases	NAC	I*	I	I*
15. As numbers supervised increase	NAC	NAC	D	D*
16. As rewards and achievement decrease	I	I*	I*	I
17. As performance falls	I	NAC	NAC	I*
18. As communications upward worsen	I*	D	I*	I*
19. As communications downward worsen	I*	I	NAC	I*
20. As conflict increases	I*	D	NAC	I*
21. As visits to the doctor increase	NAC	NAC	NAC	D
22. As lateness for work increases	I	NAC	NAC	D
23. As accidents increase	I	NAC	D	NAC
24. As absence increases	D*	I	NAC	I
25. As smoking increases	NAC	NAC	I*	NAC
26. As drink increases	NAC	NAC	I	I
27. As worry increases	I	NAC	I	I*
28. As perfectionism increases	I	NAC	I*	NAC
29. As enjoyment of work decreases	I*	I	NAC	I
30. As confidence falls	I	D*	I	NAC

Correlation Between Job Factors and Stress
* indicates a high level of correlation. NAC = No apparent correlation. I = increase. D = decrease.

Appendix B

Certified sickness absence – year ending June, 1974

Causes	Days lost at Work	
	Total for men	Total for women
Psychoses	7,018,880	2,678,480
Neuroses	12,963,880	6,111,480
Personality disorders	453,400	127,160
Mental retardation	448,240	152,080
Migraine	285,560	190,120
Hypertensive diseases	6,452,040	1,367,520
Ulcer of the duodenum	1,748,520	65,320
Peptic ulcer (site unspecified)	1,886,320	141,480
Nervousness and debility	3,705,480	3,545,160
Headaches	335,480	156,560
	35,297,800	14,535,360

Source: DHSS (totals based on 2.5 per cent sample)

INDEX

Absence, casual, 45
   sickness, 18
Accidents, 45
Aches, muscular, 23, 47, 51
Achievement, 89, 94, 97
Addiction, 46
Age, 78
Alcoholism, 19, 46, 109
Alienation, 64
Anxiety, 46, 47, 51
Appointed Factory Doctors, 116
Appraisal, 96
Assessment Panel, 122
Attitudes to work, 97

Back log, 87
Blake and Mouton, 126
Blood pressure, 46, 51
Breakdown, 36, 120, 127
British Medical Dictionary, 42
British Medical Association, 116
Brook, A., 79
Burns and Stalker, 72
Business schools, 126

C.B.I., 126
Career development, 96
Careers education, 125
Change, 64, 84
Code of Industrial Relations Practice, 117
Communication, 73, 89, 100
Community development, 62
Company policy, 107
Confidentiality, 120
Conflict, 106
Cost of stress at work, 18
Counselling, 117, 122

Department of Education and Science, 125

Department of Employment, 18, 115
   News, 19, 116
   Gazette, 86
Department of Health and Social Security, 115
Depression, 46, 47, 51
Discipline, 90, 93
Digestion, 47
Doctors, 115, 121, 127
Dread, 47
Drink, 109
Drucker, Peter, 119
Drugs, 46

Education, 104, 125
Employment Medical Advisory Service, 115, 120, 127
Energy cycle, 33
Engels, F., 64
Engineering, 36
Environment, 61
Ethics, 124
Experience, 79, 98

Factories Act, 19
Faith, 124
Family, 27, 85, 128
Fear of health breakdown, 48, 51
Fraser, R., 17
Friedmann, G., 17
Fromm, E., 65

Government, 18, 127
Grievance procedures, 108

Haemorrhage, cerebral, 42
Harvard Business Review, 94
Headaches, 24, 28, 29, 51

Index

Health and Safety at Work Act, 18, 115, 127
Heart trouble, 51
Herzberg, F., 17, 18, 20
Home, 32, 86, 110, 129
Hypertension, 47
Hysteria, 46

Indecision, 26, 30
Indigestion, 47, 51
Industrial Relations, 18, 81, 90, 108
Industrial Society, 32
International Committee on Occupational Mental Health, 48
International Labour Office, 86
Irritability, 47, 51

Jacques, E., 17
Job descriptions, 84
Job satisfaction, 123

Kearns, J. L., 42

Lateness, 93
Length of service, 79
Leisure, 70
Listening, 102, 104
Load, overload, 36
Loss of temper, 29, 47, 51

Macmillan, M., 115
MacNalty's British Medical Dictionary, 42
Managers, 30, 31, 61, 71, 94, 96, 99, 101, 117, 123, 128
Management, 31, 44, 48, 70, 71, 74, 90, 101, 105, 114, 117, 127
  Techniques, 82
  Styles, 118
Marriage, 128
Marx, K., 64
McGregor, D., 92
Mental Health, 17, 19, 111, 119
Method study, 87
Migraine, 29, 47, 51, 59

Misrepresentation, 106
Motivation, 106

Nepotism, 71
Neurosis, 46
North East England, 61

Objections, 106
Objectives, 102, 123
Occupational Medicine, 115
Office of Health Economics, 19, 46, 115
Organization, 52, 59, 72, 87, 94, 99, 108, 119, 124
Organizational development, 81, 119
Overload, 36
Overtime, 34, 86
Overwork, 47, 51

Pahl, J. J. and R. E., 128
Paperwork, 89
Parsons, 59
Participation, 117
Pay, 94
Perfectionism, 27
Performance, 44, 94, 102, 109
Personal needs, 95
Personality, 31
Personnel department, 117
Pilfering, 94
Planners, 128
Polytechnics, 126
Pressure, 36, 48, 61, 128
Problem avoidance, 108
  solving, 81, 123
Procedures, 90, 108
Procrastination, 47, 51
Production orientation, 99
Productivity, 99, 109, 127
Promotion, 75, 81, 96
Primary stress symptoms, 51, 114
Prospects, 96
Psychoneurosis, 46
Psychosis, 46
Publicity, 115

Index

Qualifications, 73, 80
Quality, 93

Rebellion, 94
Recognition, 97, 99
Recreation, 33
Relationships, 93, 106, 114
Relaxation, 33
Research, 56
Resentment, 94, 106
Resistance to change, 107
Responsibility, 91, 98
Restructuring, 94
Retired men, 59
Review, 102
Rewards, 94
Robertson, K., 117
Roben's Committee, 18, 116
Routine, 90

Saab-Scania, 94
Sabotage, 94
Safety and Health at work, 18, 116
Schilling, R. S. F., 79
School leavers, 98
Screening, 120
Secretary, 29, 102
Selection, 93, 98
Selye, H., 17, 43
Sensitivity, 28, 109
Sexual intercourse, 46
Shareholders, 127
Shift work, 26, 85, 104
Shop steward, 74, 107, 121
Shop floor, 103
Sleep, sleeplessness, 34, 47, 51, 85
Smoking, 46, 109
Social insecurity, 63
Society of Occupational Medicine, 116
Stress, analysis, 55
  cause of, 31, 35
  count, 49
  definition, 43
  feeling of, 51
  incidence, 58
  levels, 50, 55
  meaning of, 36, 43
  patterns, 56, 59
  primary symptoms, 45, 51, 61, 114
  problem, 17, 30
  scores, 53, 121
  secondary symptoms, 45, 61, 114
  stages of, 43
  symptoms, 44–49, 50, 53
  temperature, 52
Supervisor, 44, 56, 71, 111, 117, 129
Support, 110

T.U.C., 126
Teachers, 125
  student, 59
Teamwork, 98
Tension, 21, 47, 51
Thrombosis, 42, 47, 51
Timekeeping, 93
Tiredness, 47, 51
Toffler, A., 119
Trade Unions, 18, 31, 70, 73, 94, 99, 118, 123, 124, 126
Training, 74, 81, 89, 91, 97, 99, 111, 115, 116
Tolpuddle Martyrs, 124
Travel, 88
Treatment, 127
Trust, 106
Turn-over, labour, 94

Understanding, 105, 110, 128
Ulcers, 47, 51
Underemployment, 37

Volvo, 94, 118

Walton, R. E., 94
Waste, 94
Withdrawal, 32, 94
Wives, 110, 128
Work, 65
  attitudes, 98
  capacity for, 37

Work—*cont.*
 dread of going to, 47, 51, 58
 lack of interest in, 47, 51
 place, 31
 restructuring, 94

Works Medical Officers, 116
Worry, 26, 107, 109

Yielding, 36
Yieldpoint, 37